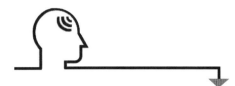

Transcranial Magnetic Stimulation

—

Clinical Applications for
Psychiatric Practice

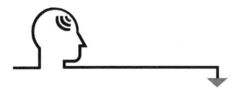

Transcranial Magnetic Stimulation

—

Clinical Applications for Psychiatric Practice

Edited by

Richard A. Bermudes, M.D.
Karl I. Lanocha, M.D.
Philip G. Janicak, M.D.

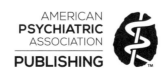

AMERICAN
PSYCHIATRIC
ASSOCIATION
PUBLISHING

If you wish to buy 50 or more copies of the same title, please go to www.appi.org/specialdiscounts for more information.

Copyright © 2018 American Psychiatric Association Publishing

ALL RIGHTS RESERVED

First Edition

Manufactured in the United States of America on acid-free paper
22   5 4 3

American Psychiatric Association Publishing
1000 Wilson Boulevard
Arlington, VA 22209-3901
www.appi.org

Library of Congress Cataloging-in-Publication Data
Names: Bermudes, Richard A., 1967- editor. | Lanocha, Karl I., editor. | Janicak, Philip G., editor. | American Psychiatric Association Publishing, issuing body.
Title: Transcranial magnetic stimulation : clinical applications for psychiatric practice / edited by Richard A. Bermudes, Karl I. Lanocha, Philip G. Janicak.
Other titles: Transcranial magnetic stimulation (Bermudes)
Description: First edition. | Arlington, VA : American Psychiatric Association Publishing, [2018] | Includes bibliographical references and index.
Identifiers: LCCN 2017035039 (print) | LCCN 2017036310 (ebook) | ISBN 9781615371716 (eb) | ISBN 9781615371051 (pb : alk. paper)
Subjects: | MESH: Transcranial Magnetic Stimulation | Depressive Disorder–therapy
Classification: LCC RC386.2 (ebook) | LCC RC386.2 (print) | NLM WM   171.5 | DDC 616.89/12–dc23
LC record available at https://lccn.loc.gov/2017035039

British Library Cataloguing in Publication Data
A CIP record is available from the British Library.

Contents

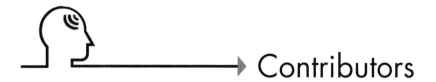

Contributors

Scott T. Aaronson, M.D.
Director, Clinical Research Programs, Sheppard Pratt Health System, Baltimore, Maryland

Sasha Bergeron, M.S.N., PMHNP-BC
Psychiatric Nurse Practitioner, TMS Health Solutions, Oakland, California

Richard A. Bermudes, M.D.
Chief Medical Officer, TMS Health Solutions; Assistant Clinical Professor-Volunteer, Department of Psychiatry, University of California, San Francisco, San Francisco, California

Ian A. Cook, M.D., DFAPA
Founding Director, UCLA TMS Clinical Service (2009–2014); Professor of Psychiatry and Biobehavioral Sciences and of Bioengineering and Chief Translational Innovational Officer, Semel Institute for Neuroscience and Human Behavior, University of California, Los Angeles; Psychiatrist, Greater Los Angeles Veterans Administration Health System, Los Angeles, California

Paul E. Croarkin, D.O., M.S.
Consultant and Associate Professor of Psychiatry, Mayo Clinic, Rochester, Minnesota

Danielle D. DeSouza, Ph.D.

Instructor, Department of Neurology and Neurological Sciences, Stanford University School of Medicine, Palo Alto, California

Mehmet E. Dokucu, M.D., Ph.D.

Associate Professor and Director, Neuromodulation Program, Department of Psychiatry and Behavioral Sciences, Northwestern University Feinberg School of Medicine, Chicago, Illinois

David L. Dunner, M.D., FACPsych

Director, Center for Anxiety and Depression, Mercer Island, Washington; Professor Emeritus, Department of Psychiatry and Behavioral Sciences, University of Washington, Seattle

Philip G. Janicak, M.D.

Adjunct Professor, Department of Psychiatry and Behavioral Sciences, Northwestern University Feinberg School of Medicine; Director, Transcranial Magnetic Stimulation Center, Linden Oaks Medical Group at Edward/Elmhurst Healthcare, Naperville, Illinois

Karl I. Lanocha, M.D.

Director of Education, TMS Health Solutions, San Francisco, California

Jaspreet Pannu, B.Sc.

Medical Student, Brain Stimulation Laboratory, Department of Psychiatry and Behavioral Sciences, Stanford University School of Medicine, Stanford, California

Kristin S. Raj, M.D.

Clinical Instructor, Department of Psychiatry and Behavioral Sciences, Stanford University School of Medicine, Stanford, California

Zoe Samara, Ph.D.

Postdoctoral Fellow, Williams PanLab, Department of Psychiatry and Behavioral Sciences, Stanford University School of Medicine, Stanford, California

Nolan R. Williams, M.D.

Director, Brain Stimulation Laboratory, Department of Psychiatry and Behavioral Sciences, Stanford University School of Medicine, Stanford, California

Disclosure of Competing Interests

The following contributors to this book have indicated a financial interest in or other affiliation with a commercial supporter, a manufacturer of a commercial product, a provider of a commercial service, a nongovernmental organization, and/or a government agency, as listed below:

Scott T. Aaronson, M.D.—*Consulting income*: LivaNova, Janssen, Genomind; *Speaker's bureau*: Sunovion, Otsuka/Lundbeck; *Research support*: Neuronetics (equipment only)

Ian A. Cook, M.D., DFAPA—Within the past 7 years, Dr. Cook has received research support from Aspect Medical Systems/Covidien, National Institutes of Health, Neuronetics, and Shire; he has been on the speaker's bureau for Neuronetics and the Medical Education Speakers Network; he has been an advisor/consultant/reviewer for Allergan, Arctica Health, Cerêve, Covidien, Pfizer, NeuroDetect, Neuronetics, NeuroSigma, NIH (ITVA), U.S. Departments of Defense and Justice, VA (DSMB); he is a past member of the editorial board of the *World Journal of Biological Psychiatry* and is Editor of the Patient Management section of the American Psychiatric Association's *FOCUS* journal; his biomedical intellectual property is assigned to the Regents of the University of California; he owns stock options in NeuroSigma, where he has served as Chief Medical Officer (on leave); he is primarily employed by the University of California, Los Angeles, and also has an appointment as a Staff Psychiatrist, TMS and Mood Disorders programs, Greater Los Angeles Veterans Administration Health System.

Paul E. Croarkin, D.O., M.S.—*Investigator-initiated grant support*: Pfizer ASPIRE Grant (WS1976243); *Grant in-kind support*: Assurex (supplies and genotyping for an investigator-initiated study) and Neuronetics (supplies for investigator-initiated studies); *Primary investigator*: Multicenter trial sponsored by Neuronetics; *Research grants*: Brain and Behavior Research Foundation, Mayo Clinic Foundation, National Institute of Mental Health (K23 MH100266).

David L. Dunner, M.D., FACPsych—*Owner*: NeuroStar TMS device; *Consultant*: McKesson and Neuronetics

Philip G. Janicak, M.D.—*Consultant* and *Speaker*: Neuronetics

The following contributors to this book have indicated no competing interests to disclose during the year preceding manuscript submission:

Sasha Bergeron, M.S.N., PMHNP-BC
Richard A. Bermudes, M.D.
Mehmet E. Dokucu, M.D., Ph.D.
Karl I. Lanocha, M.D.
Nolan R. Williams, M.D.

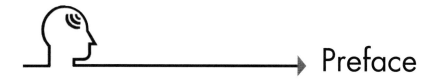

Preface

Psychiatric disorders represent a significant and growing problem for society. In addition to being a leading cause of disability worldwide (Lépine and Briley 2011; Prince et al. 2007), many of these disorders increase the risk for medical conditions such as coronary artery disease and diabetes, two leading causes of morbidity and mortality (Druss et al. 2011; Osborn et al. 2008). While many patients are effectively treated with pharmacotherapy, psychotherapy, or a combination of the two, up to 30% of patients with mood and anxiety conditions do not respond to these standard treatments (Bystritsky 2006; Rush et al. 2006).

In October 2008, the first transcranial magnetic stimulation (TMS) system was cleared by the U.S. Food and Drug Administration (FDA) for the treatment of adult patients with major depression who have not responded to one antidepressant medication. This marked the beginning of the most important treatment development for psychiatry in the last decade.

Because TMS is currently FDA cleared to treat patients with major depressive disorder, this text focuses on its clinical application for psychiatric practitioners who treat depression. In addition to the supporting literature on the efficacy and safety of TMS for depression, we also examine the ongoing research evolution of TMS as a potential treatment for other clinical neuropsychiatric conditions.

Patients have access to this ground-breaking form of neuromodulation at numerous centers in the United States. TMS therapy has an expanded FDA clearance to include adult patients with major depressive disorder who have experienced one or more failed trials of antidepressant medication. Furthermore, research is broadening to include adolescents and bipolar patients with depression as well as patients with obsessive-compulsive disorder. TMS is covered by Medicare and by all major health plans in the United States.

Despite the growing availability of this innovative option, many practitioners are unsure about how to best utilize TMS. This lack of clarity is partly because most psychiatric residency programs do not offer any curriculum on TMS therapy and continuing education conferences are limited.

This book provides mental health practitioners with a practical reference for the management of patients who are candidates for TMS. In this context, we discuss the integration of TMS with psychotherapy, pharmacotherapy, and other forms of neuromodulation; the identification of appropriate patients for referral to a TMS clinician; the coordination of care by the primary treatment team and TMS service to ensure the best outcomes during the acute, continuation, and maintenance treatment phases of depression; and the evolving nature of TMS research, such as the ongoing development of this and related technologies. The volume appendix lists a variety of options for advanced TMS training, both theoretical and hands-on, sponsored by specialty societies and medical centers.

The chapter authors are clinician-researchers with extensive knowledge about the clinical applications of TMS, as well as other forms of neuromodulation. The discussion in Chapter 1, "Transcranial Magnetic Stimulation Therapy for Treatment-Resistant Depression," covers basic principles and technology, development of TMS, an overview of parameters, efficacy, and the mechanism of action. The following chapters provide a review of the literature for a particular topic, as well as one or more clinical vignettes that highlight how TMS is integrated into patient care. Although the TMS literature has grown exponentially in the last 10 years, clinicians must still manage patients whose histories may differ from those of study populations. Therefore, each chapter also provides a list of key clinical points that summarize the optimal clinical application of TMS for the general mental health provider. In summary, this work provides both an update on the present clinical role of TMS and a road map to its potential future.

Richard A. Bermudes, M.D.
Karl I. Lanocha, M.D.
Philip G. Janicak, M.D.

References

Bystritsky A: Treatment-resistant anxiety disorders. Mol Psychiatry 11(9):805–814, 2006 16847460

Druss BG, Zhao L, Von Esenwein S, et al: Understanding excess mortality in persons with mental illness: 17-year follow up of a nationally representative US survey. Med Care 49(6):599–604, 2011 21577183

Lépine JP, Briley M: The increasing burden of depression. Neuropsychiatr Dis Treat 7 (suppl 1):3–7, 2011 21750622

Osborn DP, Wright CA, Levy G, et al: Relative risk of diabetes, dyslipidaemia, hypertension and the metabolic syndrome in people with severe mental illnesses: systematic review and metaanalysis. BMC Psychiatry 8:84, 2008 18817565

Prince M, Patel V, Saxena S, et al: No health without mental health. Lancet 370(9590):859–877, 2007 17804063

Rush AJ, Trivedi MH, Wisniewski SR, et al: Acute and longer-term outcomes in depressed outpatients requiring one or several treatment steps: a STAR*D report. Am J Psychiatry 163(11):1905–1917 2006 17074942

Transcranial Magnetic Stimulation Therapy for Treatment-Resistant Depression

Karl I. Lanocha, M.D.

Transcranial magnetic stimulation (TMS) is a safe, noninvasive neuromodulation procedure that uses high-strength pulsed magnetic fields to induce a depolarizing current in a localized area of the cerebral cortex. Introduced into research in 1985, TMS was first used experimentally to treat depression in the mid-1990s. In 2008, the U.S. Food and Drug Administration (FDA) cleared a specific TMS device for use in

---

Note. Although TMS and repetitive TMS are technically different, in this book the abbreviation TMS is used predominantly.

treating patients with unipolar major depression who had failed to respond to conventional antidepressant medication treatment.

TMS represents an important breakthrough in the treatment of depression for a variety of reasons, including the following:

- TMS is effective for patients who fail to respond to antidepressant medication.
- Unlike electroconvulsive therapy (ECT), TMS is an office-based procedure that requires no anesthesia or sedation.
- Unlike ECT, TMS causes no cognitive side effects.
- Unlike medications, TMS causes no systemic side effects such as weight gain or sexual dysfunction.
- Unlike medications, which are prone to patient error and nonadherence, TMS is an observed procedure during which the clinician can ensure proper administration.

In this chapter, I provide an overview of TMS. An explanation of the basic principles underlying the procedure is followed by a brief history of the development of TMS as a treatment for depression, a general overview of how different TMS parameters affect brain function, and a review of the efficacy of TMS in the treatment of depression, including controlled trials and naturalistic observational studies. A typical course of treatment is described along with a more detailed explanation of standard stimulus parameters and variations that may be employed. The chapter concludes with a discussion about the mechanism of action of TMS.

Basic Principles and Technology of TMS

The fundamental concepts underlying TMS have been understood for over a century. Electricity and magnetism are two aspects of the same phenomenon. Every electrical current creates a magnetic field, and a magnetic field can create an electrical field in the surrounding space. TMS is a clinical application of Faraday's law of induction, which states that a moving magnetic field causes an electrical current to flow in a nearby conductor (Faraday 1831/1965). In the case of TMS, the electrical conductor is the human brain (Figure 1–1). Thus, TMS may be considered a form of *brain electrical stimulation without the use of electrodes*.

All TMS devices share the same basic elements (Figure 1–2). A *capacitor* is used to store electricity. A *thyristor switch* is used to precisely control the flow of current. Rapidly turning the current on and off produces a time-varying or moving magnetic field as the current flows through a

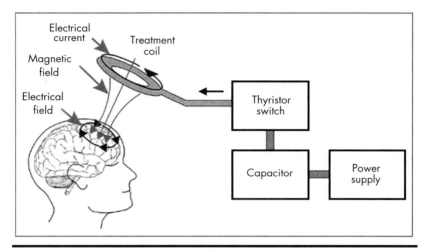

Figure 1–1.   A moving magnetic field causes electrical current to flow in nearby neural tissue.

Although not depicted in this illustration, the transcranial magnetic stimulation coil must be in direct contact with the patient's scalp to produce an electrical field strong enough to cause depolarization.

coiled cable (Davey and Epstein 2000). Peak voltages are typically on the order of 2,000 V, and currents are around 10,000 A.

The size and shape of the TMS coil determine the size and shape of the induced electrical field. TMS coils come in many shapes. The simplest, and historically the first to be used, is a *circle* measuring about 8–15 cm in diameter. Such round coils can stimulate a large area of the brain but cannot be focused. Two round coils placed side by side form what is known as a *figure-eight* or *butterfly coil*. This design allows stimulation at a limited and clearly defined location. For this reason, figure-eight coils have become the most widely used for research and therapeutic purposes (see Figure 10–1 in Chapter 10, "Current FDA-Cleared TMS Systems and Future Innovations in TMS Therapy").

Depth of penetration is limited by the laws of physics because magnetic field strength decreases exponentially as a function of distance. The magnetic field strength of TMS is approximately 1.5–2.5 teslas at the surface of the coil. This is about the same strength as a first-generation magnetic resonance imaging (MRI) machine and more than 30,000 times stronger than the earth's magnetic field, yet it is barely detectable only a few centimeters away. Most figure-eight coils activate a cortical area of approximately 2–3 cm and to a depth of approximately 2–3 cm (Deng et al. 2013). A newer type of coil, known as the *Hesed* or *H coil*, uses multi-

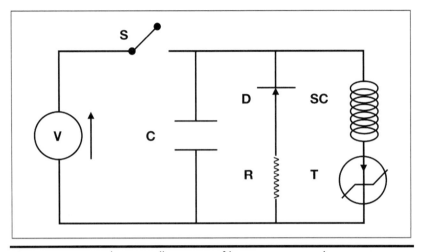

Figure 1–2. Schematic illustration of basic transcranial magnetic stimulation circuit design: capacitor, thyristor switch, and stimulating coil.

Ancillary circuits include those for temperature monitoring and for setting the frequency and intensity of pulses. C=capacitor; D=diode; R=resistance; S=switch; SC=stimulating coil; T=thyristor; V=charging circuit.

ple coil windings to achieve greater depth of penetration but with less precise focus. Basically, the deeper the penetration, the more diffuse the electrical field (see Figure 10–2 in Chapter 10).

Figure 1–3 shows an example of a TMS delivery system. Chapter 10 provides an in-depth discussion of several FDA-approved TMS delivery systems.

Development of TMS

The first magnetic nerve stimulator was built by Anthony Barker and colleagues at the University of Sheffield in 1985 (Barker et al. 1985). Although this was originally intended for peripheral nerve stimulation, it was quickly discovered that placing the coil over the motor cortex allowed for quick and easy, noninvasive stimulation of upper motor neurons.

Early TMS research focused primarily on motor cortex excitability and plasticity using single or paired pulses of TMS. These early experiments showed that magnetic stimulation could produce changes in cortical excitability lasting for a few seconds or up to several minutes (Uozumi et al. 1991). Advances in electronics soon allowed for the development of repetitive TMS, in which multiple volleys or trains of pulses at frequencies

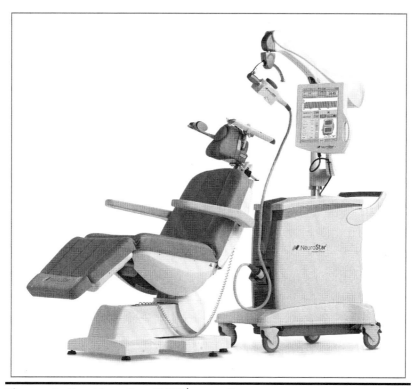

Figure 1–3. NeuroStar TMS Therapy System.

Source. Image courtesy of Neuronetics, Inc.

between 1 Hz and 50 Hz can be administered in rapid succession. (In this volume, TMS and repetitive TMS will be used interchangeably.) This technical development allowed magnetic stimulation to induce changes in cortical excitability lasting for a few minutes or up to several hours or longer.

These aftereffects are thought to be due to long-term potentiation and long-term depression mechanisms. Pioneering studies on motor cortex showed that TMS delivered at low frequencies (≤ 1 Hz) for several minutes was able to reduce the amplitude of motor evoked potentials, reflecting a decrease in cortical excitability (Chen et al. 1997). On the other hand, TMS delivered at higher frequencies (≥ 5 Hz) increased motor evoked potentials, reflecting an increase in cortical excitability (Pascual-Leone et al. 1994).

This research yielded important insights, occurring at a time when functional brain imaging studies began to shed light on the pathophysiology of psychiatric disorders. One of the most important findings from this research was *decreased left prefrontal activity in major depression*. Positron emission tomography (PET) and single-photon emission computed tomography (SPECT) studies demonstrated a correlation between the depressed state and reduced regional cerebral metabolic rate of glucose uptake and reduced regional cerebral blood flow in the left dorsolateral prefrontal cortex (DLPFC) (Mayberg 2003). Increased activity of the right prefrontal region was also demonstrated (Drevets et al. 2008). Further, functional MRI and PET studies correlated depressive behavior with hypermetabolism of the subgenual cingulate cortex and amygdala (Savitz and Drevets 2009a) and hypometabolism of the dorsal prefrontal cortex and striatal regions (Ressler and Mayberg 2007), thus defining a "depression circuit" (Figure 1–4). These developments allowed researchers to investigate the potential use of TMS as a treatment for depression by "normalizing" the activity of the left DLPFC using high-frequency, excitatory TMS (Schutter 2009) and reducing the activity of the right DLPFC using low-frequency, inhibitory TMS to restore the interhemispheric balance between left and right DLPFC activity (Schutter 2010).

General Overview of TMS Parameters

In a clinical context, TMS is usually described in terms of four separate but interrelated parameters:

- Location—brain region stimulated
- Intensity—magnetic field strength (induced electrical field strength)
- Frequency—number of pulses per second *and* frequency of treatment sessions
- Duration—number of pulses per treatment session *and* total number of treatment sessions

Together, these parameters form the basis of TMS dosage and administration.

LOCATION

The effects of TMS depend on which brain region is stimulated. For example, stimulating the motor cortex produces an immediately observable response in the form of a contralateral skeletal muscle contraction. Stimulating the occipital cortex can produce the subjective experience of flashing lights (phosphenes). Stimulating Broca's area can cause momentary speech arrest (Pascual-Leone et al. 1991). Stimulating most other cortical areas, however, produces no immediately observable or

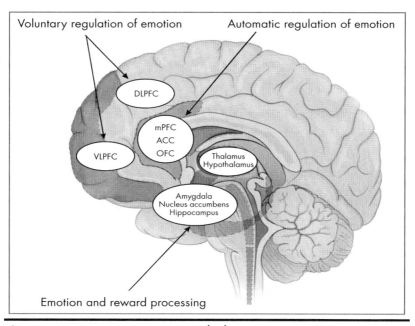

Figure 1–4. Depression circuit in the brain.

Left-sided lateral view of the brain, indicating the key structures and functions implicated in the pathophysiology of major depressive disorder: dorsolateral prefrontal cortex (DLPFC) and medial prefrontal cortex (mPFC)—executive function, regulation of emotion and assessment of consequences in decision making, and extensive connections with anterior cingulate cortex (ACC) and limbic areas, including hippocampus and amygdala; orbitofrontal cortex (OFC)—integration of multimodal stimuli and assessment of stimulus value and/or reward; ventrolateral prefrontal cortex (VLPFC)—attentional control; ACC—extensive connections with brain structures implicated in emotional behavior, key part of an extended network in emotional processing and autonomic regulation; thalamus—sensory relay, extensive connections with limbic system and mood-related circuitry; hypothalamus—linking of nervous system to endocrine system; synthesizing and secreting of neurohormones, including corticotropin releasing factor, key structure in controlling hypothalamic-pituitary adrenal axis (HPA) function; amygdala—evaluation of experience/stimuli with strong emotional valence and acquisition and expression of emotionally laden memories; nucleus accumbens—reward, pleasure, and pain avoidance; and hippocampus—learning, memory, and cognition, site of adult neurogenesis, and negative regulation of HPA axis.

subjective response. This is clearly the case with TMS treatment for depression, in that clinical results are typically seen only after several weeks of stimulation.

The most common stimulus target for treating depression is the left DLPFC.

INTENSITY

Magnetic field strength must be strong enough to induce an electrical field capable of causing depolarization. In routine clinical practice, the intensity of the transcranial magnetic stimulus is usually expressed as a percentage of the patient's *motor threshold* (MT), which is defined as the average minimum stimulus required to produce a visible muscle movement (or evoked motor potential) 50% of the time. For TMS treatment of depression, MT is usually determined by observing contractions of the right abductor pollicis brevis muscle.

> *The most common stimulus intensity for treating depression is 120% of the patient's motor threshold.*

FREQUENCY

The speed, or the number of magnetic pulses per second, determines the effect on the underlying brain tissue being stimulated. Slow pulses of 1 Hz or less decrease the excitability of the stimulus target. Frequencies greater than 1 Hz increase the excitability of the stimulus target.

> *The most common stimulus frequency for treating depression is 10 Hz.*

DURATION

Early studies of TMS treatment for depression typically involved the administration of several dozen to a few hundred pulses per treatment session. Treatment courses lasted anywhere from a few days to several weeks. Over time, the total number of pulses per treatment session and the total number of sessions in a single course of treatment steadily increased.

> *TMS treatment for depression typically involves treatment 5 days/week, Monday through Friday.*
>
> *Treatment sessions generally last 20–45 minutes.*
>
> *On average, 30 or more treatments consisting of 3,000 or more pulses per session are needed for maximum therapeutic benefit.*

Efficacy of TMS Treatment for Depression

Evidence for the clinical efficacy of TMS in the treatment of depression includes more than 30 sham-controlled clinical studies involving over 2,000 patients. Aggregate data have been examined in more than 15 meta-analyses and qualitative reviews, providing a consistent, comprehensive, and replicated literature base.

FDA REGISTRATION STUDY

FDA clearance of TMS was based on a specific treatment protocol delivered by a specific device in a large ($N=301$ patients), multisite ($N=23$), randomized sham-controlled trial (O'Reardon et al. 2007). Patients in this study had failed to respond to at least one and no more than four antidepressant medications and were medication free at the time of the study.

When this trial was designed, it was not clear how long patients needed to be treated. Many previous studies administered treatment for only 2 weeks, which is much less than is usually needed for medications (typically 6–8 weeks) or ECT (2–4 weeks) to take effect. Also unclear was the overall intensity of stimulation required. Many previous studies used stimuli of 90%–110% of MT, sometimes administering only a few hundred pulses per treatment session.

In the O'Reardon et al. (2007) study, treatment was provided 5 days/ week (Monday through Friday) for 4–6 weeks, followed by a 3-week tapering phase. Patients received up to 36 sessions of TMS therapy in 9 weeks. The treatment protocol used high-intensity, high-frequency stimulation of 10 Hz at 120% of MT delivered over the left DLPFC with 75 four-second-long pulse trains, totaling 3,000 pulses per treatment session. This duration and intensity of stimulation was unprecedented at the time.

Active TMS was found to be significantly superior to sham TMS based on patients' scores on the Montgomery-Åsberg Depression Rating Scale (MADRS) at week 4 (with a post hoc correction for inequality in symptom severity between groups at baseline), as well as on the 17- and 24-item Hamilton Depression Rating Scale (HDRS-17 and HDRS-24) at weeks 4 and 6. Response rates were significantly higher with active TMS than sham TMS on all three scales at weeks 4 and 6. Remission rates were approximately twofold higher with active TMS than sham TMS at week 6 and were significant on the MADRS and HDRS-24 (but not the HDRS-17). Active TMS was well tolerated, with a low dropout rate for adverse events (4.5%), which were generally mild and limited to transient scalp discomfort or pain (O'Reardon et al. 2007).

Patients who failed to benefit from at least 4 weeks of randomized treatment assignment in the controlled trial (either active or sham) were eligible to participate in an open-label extension trial, although patients and investigators remained blinded to prior assignment at the time of entry into this phase (Avery et al. 2008). For those patients who received sham TMS in the preceding randomized controlled trial ($N=85$), the mean reduction in MADRS scores after 6 weeks of open-label active TMS was 17.0. Furthermore, based on the MADRS, at 6 weeks, 36 of these patients (42.4%) achieved response and 17 patients (20.0%) achieved remission (i.e., MADRS score <10). For those patients who received but did not respond to active TMS in the preceding randomized controlled trial ($N=73$), the mean reduction in MADRS scores was 12.5, and response and remission rates were 26.0% and 11.0%, respectively.

OPTIMIZATION OF TMS FOR DEPRESSION STUDY

An independent (nonindustry) study sponsored by the National Institute of Mental Health (NIMH)—Optimization of TMS for Depression (OPT-TMS)—corroborated the results of the FDA registration study. This NIMH study used the same device and same treatment parameters as the FDA study but with several methodological improvements, including MRI adjustment for coil placement, an adaptive flexible duration of treatment, an improved sham device that better mimicked the sensory experience of TMS, and continuous assessment of outcome evaluator reliability relative to a masked external expert rater (George et al. 2010). High-intensity TMS for at least 3 weeks was found to be significantly more likely than sham TMS to induce remission (the primary end point) in antidepressant medication–free patients with moderately treatment-resistant unipolar major depressive disorder. It should be noted that the level of treatment resistance in this study was higher than in the FDA registration study.

DEEP TMS STUDY

The coil (H coil) used in deep TMS is able to modulate cortical excitability up to a maximum depth of 6 cm and is therefore able not only to modulate the activity of the cerebral cortex but also the activity of deeper neural circuits (Bersani et al. 2013).

The Brainsway Deep TMS System H1 coil device was cleared by the FDA in 2013. The intent-to-treat sample included 212 patients at 20 sites in four different countries. All patients had failed to respond to trials of one to four antidepressant medications during the current episode and were randomly assigned to receive either active deep TMS or sham treatment. Patients, treaters, and raters were fully blinded. A total of 181 patients completed the study per protocol. Acute treatment consisted of five sessions per week for 4 weeks, followed by a continuation phase of twice-weekly treatment for 12 more weeks. The stimulation site was the left DLPFC, although broader stimulation is likely with the H1 coil. Stimulation parameters were MT of 120%, frequency of 18 Hz, train duration of 2 seconds, intertrain interval of 20 seconds, and 55 trains per session, for a total of 1,980 pulses over 20 minutes (Levkovitz et al. 2015).

The primary end point in the Levkovitz et al. (2015) study was the change in total score on the 21-item Hamilton Depression Rating Scale (HDRS-21) from baseline to week 5. The secondary efficacy end points were response and remission rates at week 5. Response was defined as a reduction of at least 50% in the total HDRS-21 score compared with baseline, and remission was defined by a total HDRS-21 score that was lower than 10.

In the intent-to-treat sample, the difference of −2.23 points (95% confidence interval [CI]: −4.54, 0.07) between the slopes across 5 weeks fell just short of reaching statistical significance ($P=0.0578$). However, the study results were analyzed for a subset of patients who received the prescribed stimulation protocol at 120% of MT ($n=181$; 89 in the deep TMS sample and 92 in the sham sample). In this subsample of patients, the difference of −3.11 points (95% CI: −5.40, −0.83) between the slopes was statistically significant ($P=0.008$), with an effect size of 0.76.

In terms of the secondary outcome measures, at week 5, the response rates (prescribed stimulation protocol set) were 38.4% for active treatment versus 21.4% for sham TMS ($P=0.0138$), and remission rates (prescribed stimulation protocol set) were 32.6% for active treatment versus 14.6% for sham TMS ($P=0.0051$). At week 16, the response rates were 44.3% for active treatment versus 25.6% for sham TMS ($P=0.0086$), and remission rates were 31.8% for active treatment versus 22.2% for sham TMS ($P=0.1492$).

Although these response and remission rates are higher than in the previously discussed FDA registration trial and OPT-TMS study, the study populations were different, as were the primary outcome measures. Direct comparisons of deep TMS versus standard figure-eight coil TMS have yet to be done.

Naturalistic Observational Studies

In addition to the randomized controlled studies described in the previous section, several multisite, naturalistic observational studies have examined the safety and long-term effectiveness of TMS in clinical populations.

These latter studies are important because they more accurately reflect the administration of TMS in a "real-world" setting. For example, both the FDA registration study and the OPT-TMS study excluded patients with Axis I disorders other than major depression (except for simple phobia and nicotine addiction). In typical clinical practice, however, many patients receiving TMS have comorbid psychiatric illness such as an eating disorder or posttraumatic stress disorder or a history of psychosis. Similarly, in both the FDA registration study and the OPT-TMS study, patients were required to be medication free for 1 week prior to the start of the study. This is almost never the case in the real world, where virtually all patients with depression are taking one or more psychotropic medications, often from different classes.

OVERALL EFFECTIVENESS

Carpenter et al. (2012) looked at outcomes for 307 patients treated at 42 clinical TMS practice sites in the United States. The majority of patients were treated using the standard FDA-approved protocol associated with the NeuroStar device (Figure 1–3). The clinician-assessed response rate based on the Clinical Global Impression—Severity of Illness Scale (CGI-S) was 58.0% and the remission rate was 37.1%. Patient-reported response rates ranged from 56.4% to 41.5%, and remission rates ranged from 28.7% to 26.5%, based on the 9-item Patient Health Questionnaire (PHQ-9) and Inventory of Depressive Symptomatology—Self Report (IDS-SR), respectively. Overall, these outcomes were similar to those seen in research populations.

QUALITY-OF-LIFE MEASURES

Functional status and quality-of-life outcomes were also assessed in this same group of 307 patients (Janicak et al. 2013). Following acute TMS treatment, statistically significant improvement was observed in functional status on a broad range of mental health and physical health domains, based on the Medical Outcomes Study 36-item Short-Form Health Survey (SF-36). Similarly, statistically significant improvement in patient-reported quality of life was observed on all domains of the EuroQol 5-Dimensions questionnaire (EQ-5D) and on the General Health Perception and Health Index subscale scores. Improvement on these measures was observed across the entire range of baseline depression symptom severity, demonstrating that TMS as administered in routine clinical practice settings produces statistically and clinically meaningful improvements in patient-reported quality of life and functional status.

DURABILITY OF EFFECT

The durability of TMS effect following acute treatment has been demonstrated in several studies both with and without maintenance antidepressant medication. In general, these studies demonstrate high durability for acute TMS benefits. Details regarding long-term outcome studies are provided in Chapter 6, "Managing Patients After Transcranial Magnetic Stimulation."

META-ANALYTIC STUDIES

More than a dozen meta-analyses of TMS treatment of depression have been published. Schutter (2009) evaluated 30 double-blind, sham-controlled studies involving 1,164 patients and found that high-frequency TMS over the left DLPFC was superior to sham TMS, with an effect size comparable to that of commercially available antidepressant drugs. In a larger study, Slotema et al. (2010) examined 34 sham-controlled studies involving 1,383 patients; the authors concluded that TMS is effective in treating depression and has a mild side-effect profile. In a more recent meta-analysis, Gaynes et al. (2014) concluded that TMS is a reasonable and effective consideration for patients with major depression who have had at least two previous antidepressant treatment failures and that patients receiving TMS were at least five times as likely to achieve remission as patients receiving sham TMS.

TMS Treatment Parameters for Depression

STIMULUS FREQUENCY

The most common form of TMS treatment for depression involves high-frequency stimulation over the left DLPFC. A frequency of 10 Hz was used in the pivotal trials leading to FDA clearance of TMS in the United States and is the most commonly used frequency for figure-eight coil TMS. The Brainsway H1 coil stimulates at a frequency of 18 Hz. There is also a body of evidence to support the efficacy of low-frequency 1-Hz stimulation over the right DLPFC (Isenberg et al. 2005; Pallanti et al. 2010), and sequential administration of both left-sided high-frequency TMS and right-sided low-frequency TMS in the same treatment session has been used to maximize treatment efficacy (Fitzgerald et al. 2006).

A recent systematic review and network meta-analysis involving 81 studies with 4,233 patients found few differences in clinical efficacy between these different modalities (Brunoni et al. 2017).

Theta-burst stimulation (TBS) is a modified form of TMS in which a three-pulse 50-Hz burst is applied at 5 Hz (every 200 milliseconds) representing the theta rhythm. In intermittent TBS, a 2-second train of TBS is delivered every 10 seconds for 600 pulses in total. Continuous TBS involves an uninterrupted 40-second train of TBS amounting to a total of 600 pulses (Daskalakis 2014). Intermittent TBS produces long-term potentiation-like (excitatory) effects, whereas continuous TBS produces a long-term depression-like reduction of cortical excitability. These neuroplastic changes may occur within seconds (Huang et al. 2005).

Intermittent TBS is thought to increase and continuous TBS is thought to decrease the postsynaptic concentration of calcium ions, an important factor in enhancing synaptic plasticity (Huang et al. 2011). Intermittent TBS applied to the left DLPFC or a combination of intermittent TBS applied to the left DLPFC plus continuous TBS applied to the right DLPFC has been shown to be effective in treatment-resistant depression (Li et al. 2014). TBS is still considered to be investigational.

STIMULUS INTENSITY

Early TMS studies used stimulus intensities of 80%–90% of MT and generated mixed results. It eventually became clear that suprathreshold stimulation at 110%–120% of MT was necessary to produce antidepressant effects. MT is typically expressed as a percentage of the total output of the specific TMS device being used. MT is relatively stable over time and usually needs to be determined only once, at the start of treatment.

TREATMENT SITE LOCATION

Several methods may be used to determine the correct stimulation site.

Five-Centimeter Rule

The most commonly used method for determining the coil placement site involves isolating the motor cortex area corresponding to the abductor pollicis brevis muscle and moving the coil 5 cm anteriorly. This so-called 5-cm rule has been used since the 1990s and was used in the pivotal trial leading to FDA clearance. This proves that the method can be used to administer effective treatment. Studies have shown, however, that this method may result in accurate placement only about 70% of the time (Johnson et al. 2013), raising the question of whether more robust response and remission rates might be seen if coil placement could be better ensured.

The chief drawback to the 5-cm rule is that it fails to account for differences in head size and may result in the coil being placed too far posteriorly or medially. One study estimated that the 5-cm rule would localize to the premotor cortex for 32% of patients, with variable positioning for the rest (Herwig et al. 2001). Apart from the possibility of providing ineffective treatment, seizure risk may also be increased if the coil is too close to the motor cortex. Because of these concerns, some clinicians routinely position the coil forward by 1 cm or more, although moving the coil too far forward increases the likelihood of ocular pain or facial discomfort (due to stimulation of the trigeminal nerve) during treatment.

Neuronavigation

The most accurate method of treatment site location involves the use of a neuronavigation system composed of a reference MRI brain scan, stereotactic sensors, and sophisticated software to guide coil placement (Schönfeldt-Lecuona et al. 2010). It is worth noting that this method was used for about one-third of patients in the OPT-TMS trial. The chief drawbacks are the added cost and the fact that most systems are cumbersome, are difficult to use, and require a considerable amount of staff training. For these reasons, neuronavigation is rarely used outside of academic research settings where it may be essential for other TMS applications, such as treatment for stroke.

Electroencephalogram F3 Method

More accurate than the 5-cm rule and of comparable accuracy to neuronavigation is the use of the International 10-20 System of electroencephalogram electrode placement. Using this method, the target is the F3 electroencephalogram site, which corresponds to the DLPFC. Normally, this is a derived location obtained only after first taking a series of painstaking measurements. Beam et al. (2009) at the Medical University of South Carolina developed a streamlined method of locating F3 that requires only three simple measurements: tragus to tragus, nasion to inion, and head circumference. Entering these measurements into an equation yields a set of coordinates that can be easily marked on the patient's scalp, directly corresponding to F3. This method has been compared with neuronavigation and found comparable to within 3 mm (Mir-Moghtadaei et al. 2015). Table 1–1 summarizes the treatment parameters that are commonly used for treating depression.

Typical Course of Treatment

MOTOR THRESHOLD DETERMINATION AND INITIAL TREATMENT

MT determination and coil placement are essential elements of correct TMS dosage and must be determined by the treating physician. Respon-

Table 1–1. Transcranial magnetic stimulation: common stimulus parameters for major depressive disorder

Parameter	Comment
Coil location	Most often: left DLPFC
	Less often: right DLPFC
MT	Lowest stimulus intensity over primary motor cortex to produce contraction of the abductor pollicis brevis muscle, assessed visually or by electromyography
Stimulus pulse	
Intensity	90%–120% of MT
Frequency	HF 10–20 Hz; LF ≤1 Hz; TBS 3 pulses at 50 Hz
Pulse train duration	HF 2–4 seconds; LF 5–26 minutes; TBS 40–90 seconds
Pulse train interval	HF 10–28 seconds; LF 0 seconds
Number of pulses	
HF: per session	1,500–6,000
per course	Up to 216,000
LF: per session	900–1,600
per course	Up to 57,600

Note. DLPFC=dorsolateral prefrontal cortex; HF=high frequency; LF=low frequency; MT=motor threshold; TBS=theta-burst stimulation.
Source. Adapted from Janicak and Dokucu 2015.

sibility cannot be delegated to a technician or other assistant no matter how well trained. These and other best practice guidelines are contained in the "Clinical TMS Society Consensus Review and Treatment Recommendations for TMS Therapy for Major Depressive Disorder" (Perera et al. 2016).

ACUTE TREATMENT PHASE

A typical course of TMS can last 6 weeks or more. Most patients require 30–36 treatments to achieve maximum therapeutic benefit. Treatments are usually administered 5 days/week, but at least two studies have shown that overall outcome is the same when treatments are administered 3 days/week in a treatment course that is correspondingly longer (Galletly et al. 2012; Turnier-Shea et al. 2006). There is no evidence that administering treatment 7 days/week hastens recovery or produces a better outcome. One study suggests that the overall length of treatment may be shortened by administering multiple treatments over several days, without any increase in risk (Holtzheimer et al. 2010). Another study found that three TMS treatments per day over the course of 3 days brought about a rapid decrease in suicidal ideation (George et al. 2014).

A typical treatment session lasts 20–45 minutes depending on the treatment parameters used. Most patients adapt quickly to the stimulus sensation, and premature discontinuation of treatment is uncommon. The structure provided by daily treatment and the interpersonal context of treatment may have therapeutic value for some patients and are worthy of further study.

Improvement occurs gradually and is similar to the time course seen with antidepressant medication. Most patients notice improvement between 15 and 20 treatments, although earlier and later responses may occur. Core somatic symptoms typically improve before subjective sadness and other psychological symptoms do, and family or friends may notice changes first. Interestingly, many patients report a change in visual perception and find that colors appear more vivid. Many also report improved clarity of thinking and improved memory.

Regular follow-up by the treating physician is essential. Standardized rating scales such as the PHQ-9 and Quick Inventory of Depressive Symptomatology (QIDS) provide quantifiable measures of symptom severity, and their use is routinely required by many insurance plans to justify the ongoing need for treatment.

TAPERING PHASE

Although a course of TMS may sometimes end abruptly, more often it is tapered over several weeks. Typically, a course of treatment will consist of about 25–30 treatments administered 5 days/week followed by a tapering phase of three treatments for 1 week, two treatments the next week, and one treatment the final week.

Mechanism of Action

Since the monoamine hypothesis was first proposed more than 50 years ago (Schildkraut 1965), theories about the pathogenesis of depression and the mechanism of action of antidepressant medications have focused on the level of cell-to-cell interaction and synaptic transmission, with particular attention to serotonin, dopamine, and norepinephrine. Most antidepressant medications increase extracellular levels of these monoamine neurotransmitters and thereby alter synaptic signaling (Tanti and Belzung 2010).

Animal experiments have shown that prefrontal TMS affects neurotransmitter concentrations in a variety of brain regions distant from the stimulation site, including serotonin and dopamine in the prefrontal cortex, striatum, and hippocampus (Gur et al. 2000; Pogarell et al. 2007). Like antidepressants, TMS appears to normalize the function of the hypothalamic-pituitary-adrenal axis and appears to decrease corticotropin-releasing hormone (CRH) and adrenocorticotropic hormone (ACTH) (Keck et al. 2001). TMS also appears to exert a neuroprotective effect by decreasing oxidative stress (Post et al. 1999) and by increasing the level of brain-derived neurotrophic factor in the dentate gyrus of the hippocampus (Tardito et al. 2006).

Evidence suggests that enhanced neuroplasticity is a common feature of all antidepressant medications, as well as of neuromodulation treatments such as TMS (Krishnan and Nestler 2010; Racagni and Popoli 2008). In contrast to medication, however, TMS is delivered at a very different level of brain organization. Rather than targeting synaptic proteins, TMS is applied to cortical circuits.

Functional brain imaging has shown that depression is marked by dysfunction in a number of cortical regions, such as the DLPFC and anterior cingulate cortex, as well as in deep gray matter structures, including the amygdala, nucleus accumbens, and thalamic and hypothalamic nuclei. Depression is increasingly understood as a disorder of connectivity in neural networks linking these regions (Greicius et al. 2007; Leuchter et al. 2012). Many of the mood and neurovegetative symptoms, as well as deficits in cognition and memory, are thought to arise from dysfunction in networks linking cortical and subcortical gray structures (Ottowitz et al. 2002; Savitz and Drevets 2009b). Thus, major depressive disorder has been conceptualized as a syndrome of "thalamocortical dysrhythmia," marked by persistent resonance of rhythmic thalamocortical activity (Leuchter et al. 2015).

TMS may directly modulate this rhythmic thalamocortical activity in a top-down fashion at the level of large-scale networks to influence neuronal firing rates, firing patterns, and other processes at the cellular level. Conversely, medications would appear to act in a bottom-up fashion by inducing changes at the level of the synapse followed by changes in neuronal firing rates and patterns, eventually affecting network activity (Leuchter et al. 2015).

Conclusion

TMS represents a major advance in noninvasive therapeutic neuromodulation with proven efficacy in the treatment of major depressive disorder. Its safety and benign side-effect profile make it a viable treatment alternative for patients who do not respond to standard treatments. Modifications in TMS technique and improvements in TMS technology, including the development of new stimulation coils, may further enhance clinical efficacy. Research also suggests that other cortical sites, such as the ventromedial prefrontal cortex, may eventually become therapeutic targets.

While the mechanism of action of TMS is not fully understood, evidence suggests that its therapeutic effects are the result of neuroplastic changes in thalamocortical circuits involved in the expression of core symptoms of major depression. These findings, together with those derived from other lines of research, such as neuroimaging, may shed light on the pathophysiology and circuit dysfunction associated with other neuropsychiatric disorders perhaps leading to clinical applications beyond major depressive disorder.

KEY CLINICAL POINTS

- TMS is an effective treatment for patients who fail to respond to antidepressant medication and psychotherapy.

- The most common stimulus target for treating depression is the left dorsolateral prefrontal cortex, the most common stimulus intensity is 120% of the patient's motor threshold, and the most common frequency is 10 Hz. TMS treatment for depression typically involves daily treatment sessions, Monday through Friday, lasting 20–45 minutes.

- Clinical improvement may be seen in 2–3 weeks but typically requires 30 or more treatments over 4–6 weeks.

References

Avery DH, Isenberg KE, Sampson SM, et al: Transcranial magnetic stimulation in the acute treatment of major depressive disorder: clinical response in an open-label extension trial. J Clin Psychiatry 69(3):441–451, 2008 18294022

Barker AT, Jalinous R, Freeston IL: Non-invasive magnetic stimulation of human motor cortex. Lancet 1(8437):1106–1107, 1985 2860322

Beam W, Borckardt JJ, Reeves ST, et al: An efficient and accurate new method for locating the F3 position for prefrontal TMS applications. Brain Stimul 2(1):50–54, 2009 20539835

Bersani FS, Minichino A, Enticott PG, et al: Deep transcranial magnetic stimulation as a treatment for psychiatric disorders: A comprehensive review. Eur Psychiatry 28(1):30–39 2013 22559998

Brunoni AR, Chaimani A, Moffa AH, et al: Repetitive transcranial magnetic stimulation for the acute treatment of major depressive episodes: a systematic review with network meta-analysis. JAMA Psychiatry 74(2):143–152, 2017 28030740

Carpenter LL, Janicak PG, Aaronson ST, et al: Transcranial magnetic stimulation (TMS) for major depression: a multisite, naturalistic, observational study of acute treatment outcomes in clinical practice. Depress Anxiety 29(7):587–596, 2012 22689344

Chen R, Classen J, Gerloff C, et al: Depression of motor cortex excitability by low-frequency transcranial magnetic stimulation. Neurology 48(5):1398–1403, 1997 9153480

Daskalakis ZJ: Theta-burst transcranial magnetic stimulation in depression: when less may be more. Brain 137(Pt 7):1860–1862 2014 24833712

Davey K, Epstein CM: Magnetic stimulation coil and circuit design. IEEE Trans Biomed Eng 47(11):1493–1499, 2000 11077743

Deng ZD, Lisanby SH, Peterchev AV: Electric field depth-focality tradeoff in transcranial magnetic stimulation: simulation comparison of 50 coil designs. Brain Stimul 6(1):1–13, 2013 22483681

Drevets WC, Price JL, Furey ML: Brain structural and functional abnormalities in mood disorders: implications for neurocircuitry models of depression. Brain Struct Funct 213(1–2):93–118, 2008 18704495

Faraday M: Effects on the production of electricity from magnetism (1831), in Michael Faraday. Edited by Williams LP. New York, Basic Books (Chapman Hill), 1965, p 531

Fitzgerald PB, Benitez J, de Castella A, et al: A randomized, controlled trial of sequential bilateral repetitive transcranial magnetic stimulation for treatment-resistant depression. Am J Psychiatry 163(1):88–94, 2006 16390894

Galletly C, Gill S, Clarke P, et al: A randomized trial comparing transcranial magnetic stimulation given 3 days/week and 5 days/week for the treatment of major depression: is efficacy related to the duration of treatment or the number of treatments? Psychol Med 42(5):981–988, 2012 21910937

Gaynes BN, Lloyd SW, Lux L, et al: Repetitive transcranial magnetic stimulation for treatment-resistant depression: a systematic review and meta-analysis. J Clin Psychiatry 75(5):477–489, quiz 489, 2014 24922485

George MS, Lisanby SH, Avery D, et al: Daily left prefrontal transcranial magnetic stimulation therapy for major depressive disorder: a sham-controlled randomized trial. Arch Gen Psychiatry 67(5):507–516, 2010 20439832

George MS, Raman R, Benedek DM, et al: A two-site pilot randomized 3-day trial of high dose left prefrontal repetitive transcranial magnetic stimulation (rTMS) for suicidal inpatients. Brain Stimul 7(3):421–431, 2014 24731434

Greicius MD, Flores BH, Menon V, et al: Resting-state functional connectivity in major depression: abnormally increased contributions from subgenual cingulate cortex and thalamus. Biol Psychiatry 62(5):429–437, 2007 17210143

Gur E, Lerer B, Dremencov E, et al: Chronic repetitive transcranial magnetic stimulation induces subsensitivity of presynaptic serotonergic autoreceptor activity in rat brain. Neuroreport 11(13):2925–2929, 2000 11006967

Herwig U, Padberg F, Unger J, et al: Transcranial magnetic stimulation in therapy studies: examination of the reliability of "standard" coil positioning by neuronavigation. Biol Psychiatry 50(1):58–61, 2001 11457424

Holtzheimer PE III, McDonald WM, Mufti M, et al: Accelerated repetitive transcranial magnetic stimulation for treatment-resistant depression. Depress Anxiety 27(10):960–963, 2010 20734360

Huang YZ, Edwards MJ, Rounis E, et al: Theta burst stimulation of the human motor cortex. Neuron 45(2):201–206 2005 15664172

Huang YZ, Rothwell JC, Chen RS, et al: The theoretical model of theta burst form of repetitive transcranial magnetic stimulation Clin Neurophysiol 122(5):1008–1018 2011 20869307

Isenberg K, Downs D, Pierce K, et al: Low frequency rTMS stimulation of the right frontal cortex is as effective as high frequency rTMS stimulation of the left frontal cortex for antidepressant-free, treatment-resistant depressed patients. Ann Clin Psychiatry 17(3):153–159, 2005 16433057

Janicak PG, Dokucu ME: Transcranial magnetic stimulation for the treatment of major depression. Neuropsychiatr Dis Treat 11:1549–1560, 2015 26170668

Janicak PG, Dunner DL, Aaronson ST, et al: Transcranial magnetic stimulation (TMS) for major depression: a multisite, naturalistic, observational study of quality of life outcome measures in clinical practice. CNS Spectr 18(6):322–332, 2013 23895940

Johnson KA, Baig M, Ramsey D, et al: Prefrontal rTMS for treating depression: location and intensity results from the OPT-TMS multi-site clinical trial. Brain Stimul 6(2):108–117, 2013 22465743

Keck ME, Welt T, Post A, et al: Neuroendocrine and behavioral effects of repetitive transcranial magnetic stimulation in a psychopathological animal model are suggestive of antidepressant-like effects. Neuropsychopharmacology 24(4):337–349, 2001 11182529

Krishnan V, Nestler EJ: Linking molecules to mood: new insight into the biology of depression. Am J Psychiatry 167(11):1305–1320, 2010 20843874

Leuchter AF, Cook IA, Hunter AM, et al: Resting-state quantitative electroencephalography reveals increased neurophysiologic connectivity in depression. PLoS One 7(2):e32508, 2012 22384265

Leuchter AF, Hunter AM, Krantz DE, et al: Rhythms and blues: modulation of oscillatory synchrony and the mechanism of action of antidepressant treatments. Ann NY Acad Sci 1344(1):78–91, 2015 25809789

Levkovitz Y, Isserles M, Padberg F, et al: Efficacy and safety of deep transcranial magnetic stimulation for major depression: a prospective multicenter randomized controlled trial. World Psychiatry 14(1):64–73, 2015 25655160

Li CT, Chen MH, Juan CH, et al: Efficacy of prefrontal theta-burst stimulation in refractory depression: a randomized sham-controlled study. 137(Pt 7):2088–2098 2014 24817188

Mayberg HS: Modulating dysfunctional limbic-cortical circuits in depression: towards development of brain-based algorithms for diagnosis and optimised treatment. Br Med Bull 65(1):193–207, 2003 12697626

Mir-Moghtadaei A, Caballero R, Fried P, et al: Concordance between BeamF3 and MRI-neuronavigated target sites for repetitive transcranial magnetic stimulation of the left dorsolateral prefrontal cortex. Brain Stimul 8(5):965–973, 2015 26115776

O'Reardon JP, Solvason HB, Janicak PG, et al: Efficacy and safety of transcranial magnetic stimulation in the acute treatment of major depression: a multisite randomized controlled trial. Biol Psychiatry 62(11):1208–1216, 2007 17573044

Ottowitz WE, Dougherty DD, Savage CR: The neural network basis for abnormalities of attention and executive function in major depressive disorder: implications for application of the medical disease model to psychiatric disorders. Harv Rev Psychiatry 10(2):86–99, 2002 11897749

Pallanti S, Bernardi S, Di Rollo A, et al: Unilateral low frequency versus sequential bilateral repetitive transcranial magnetic stimulation: is simpler better for treatment of resistant depression? Neuroscience 167(2):323–328, 2010 20144692

Pascual-Leone A, Gates JR, Dhuna A: Induction of speech arrest and counting errors with rapid-rate transcranial magnetic stimulation. Neurology 41(5):697–702, 1991 2027485

Pascual-Leone A, Valls-Solé J, Wassermann EM, et al: Responses to rapid-rate transcranial magnetic stimulation of the human motor cortex. Brain 117 (Pt 4):847–858, 1994 7922470

Perera T, George MS, Grammer G, et al: The Clinical TMS Society Consensus Review and Treatment Recommendations for TMS Therapy for Major Depressive Disorder. Brain Stimul 9(3):336–346, 2016 27090022

Pogarell O, Koch W, Pöpperl G, et al: Acute prefrontal rTMS increases striatal dopamine to a similar degree as D-amphetamine. Psychiatry Res 156(3):251–255, 2007 17993266

Post A, Müller MB, Engelmann M, et al: Repetitive transcranial magnetic stimulation in rats: evidence for a neuroprotective effect in vitro and in vivo. Eur J Neurosci 11(9):3247–3254, 1999 10510188

Racagni G, Popoli M: Cellular and molecular mechanisms in the long-term action of antidepressants. Dialogues Clin Neurosci 10(4):385–400, 2008 19170396

Ressler KJ, Mayberg HS: Targeting abnormal neural circuits in mood and anxiety disorders: from the laboratory to the clinic. Nat Neurosci 10(9):1116–1124, 2007 17726478

Savitz J, Drevets WC: Bipolar and major depressive disorder: neuroimaging the developmental-degenerative divide. 33(5):699–771 2009a 19428491

Savitz JB, Drevets WC: Imaging phenotypes of major depressive disorder: genetic correlates. Neuroscience 164(1):300–330, 2009b 19358877

Schildkraut JJ: The catecholamine hypothesis of affective disorders: a review of supporting evidence. Am J Psychiatry 122(5):509–522, 1965 5319766

Schönfeldt-Lecuona C, Lefaucheur J-P, Cardenas-Morales L, et al: The value of neuronavigated rTMS for the treatment of depression. Neurophysiol Clin 40(1):37–43, 2010 20230934

Schutter DJ: Antidepressant efficacy of high-frequency transcranial magnetic stimulation over the left dorsolateral prefrontal cortex in double-blind sham-controlled designs: a meta-analysis. Psychol Med 39(1):65–75, 2009 18447962

Schutter DJ: Quantitative review of the efficacy of slow-frequency magnetic brain stimulation in major depressive disorder. Psychol Med 40(11):1789–1795, 2010 20102670

Slotema CW, Blom JD, Hoek HW, et al: Should we expand the toolbox of psychiatric treatment methods to include repetitive transcranial magnetic stimulation (rTMS)? A meta-analysis of the efficacy of rTMS in psychiatric disorders. J Clin Psychiatry 71(7):873–884, 2010 20361902

Tanti A, Belzung C: Open questions in current models of antidepressant action. Br J Pharmacol 159(6):1187–1200, 2010 20132212

Tardito D, Perez J, Tiraboschi E, et al: Signaling pathways regulating gene expression, neuroplasticity, and neurotrophic mechanisms in the action of antidepressants: a critical overview. Pharmacol Rev 58(1):115–134, 2006 16507885

Turnier-Shea Y, Bruno R, Pridmore S: Daily and spaced treatment with transcranial magnetic stimulation in major depression: a pilot study. Aust N Z J Psychiatry 40(9):759–763, 2006 16911750

Uozumi T, Tsuji S, Murai Y: Motor potentials evoked by magnetic stimulation of the motor cortex in normal subjects and patients with motor disorders. Electroencephalogr Clin Neurophysiol 81(4):251–256, 1991 1714818

Clinical Applications and Patient Selection

Who Should Be Referred for Transcranial Magnetic Stimulation Therapy?

Karl I. Lanocha, M.D.
Richard A. Bermudes, M.D.
Philip G. Janicak, M.D.

More than 15 million people in the United States have some form of depression (Substance Abuse and Mental Health Services Administration 2016). Less than half ever seek treatment (Pratt and Brody 2014), and 75% of those who do are managed by their primary care physician (Goldman et al. 1999). Of those who are treated, only about half receive adequate treatment (Katon et al. 1992), and far fewer receive optimal treatment. Even with optimal treatment, however, full recovery from depression is surprisingly difficult to achieve considering that there are more than 30 antidepressant medications approved by the U.S. Food and Drug Administration (FDA), as well as several evidence-based psychotherapies and augmentation agents.

The largest and most important study to date of antidepressant efficacy is the National Institute of Mental Health–sponsored Sequenced Treatment Alternatives to Relieve Depression (STAR*D) study (Rush 2007). This seminaturalistic study took 7 years to complete and involved 4,040 patients at 23 psychiatric and 18 primary care "real-world" settings. An important finding was that only 35% of properly treated patients achieved remission with the first antidepressant (i.e., citalopram) prescribed. The likelihood of achieving remission decreased steadily with each subsequent treatment failure, so that after a patient experienced three failed trials of antidepressants, the likelihood of achieving remission with additional medication trials was only about 10% (Warden et al. 2007). Despite aggressive treatment, up to 30% of patients remain symptomatic. These are patients with treatment-resistant depression.

Defining Treatment-Resistant Depression

Treatment-resistant depression (TRD) is an ambiguous term for which there is no universally agreed-upon definition; various criteria have been proposed. Table 2–1 lists common definitions of TRD. In this book, we consider TRD as the failure to achieve remission after two adequate antidepressant treatment courses with evidence-based doses and durations.

Selecting Patients for TMS

It is difficult to specify the "ideal patient" for transcranial magnetic stimulation (TMS). Response to TMS is not reliably predicted by any identified biological markers or clinical factors, such as age, sex, duration of illness, or symptom severity (Lisanby et al. 2009), and the only firm contraindication to TMS is the presence of a ferromagnetically sensitive foreign object in the head area (see Chapter 3, "Risk Management Issues in Transcranial Magnetic Stimulation for Treatment of Major Depression").

According to FDA product labeling, TMS may be considered for a patient who does not respond to any number of antidepressant treatment

Table 2–1. Common definitions of treatment-resistant depression

Posttreatment decrease in a depression rating scale score of less than 50% from pretreatment baseline

Posttreatment depression rating scale score remains higher than an established cutoff value after a specified length of treatment

Failure to achieve remission after one, two, or three adequate treatment courses

Evidence of clinical response but failure to regain functional performance

Some combination of the above

Source. Adapted from Greden JF, Riba MB, McInnis MG, Sen S: "Treatment Resistant Depression," in *Treatment Resistant Depression: A Roadmap for Effective Care*. Edited by Greden JF, Riba MB, McInnis MG. Washington, DC, American Psychiatric Publishing, 2011, p. 3. Copyright ©2011 American Psychiatric Publishing. Used with permission.

courses. TMS should be considered for all patients with TRD and not as a treatment of last resort, because it is likely to be more effective when administered earlier in the course of illness before more severe treatment resistance emerges. Table 2–2 lists key clinical factors to keep in mind when considering TMS as an option for TRD.

CLINICAL VIGNETTE

The patient is a 26-year-old single woman who was studying abroad. She had an episode of depression 6 years earlier, but she was in remission taking fluoxetine 20 mg/day until she became symptomatic approximately 3 months before returning to the United States for a brief family visit. She contacted her former psychiatrist, who referred her for TMS evaluation. Her Quick Inventory of Depressive Symptomatology—Self-Report (QIDS-SR) score of 14 showed the presence of moderate symptoms, with prolonged sleep latency, sleep fragmentation, decreased energy, and low self-esteem. She was deemed to be an appropriate candidate for TMS but was scheduled to resume her studies only 4 weeks after she was seen in consultation. Thirty left-sided high-frequency (10 Hz) dorsolateral prefrontal cortex (DLPFC) TMS treatments were administered over the course of 4 weeks, with two treatments per day administered on several days. Upon completion of treatment, her QIDS-SR score of 4 indicated that she was in remission. She was advised to continue taking fluoxetine and resumed her studies without interruption.

In the pivotal study leading to FDA clearance of TMS, patients met diagnostic criteria for recurrent, unipolar, nonpsychotic major depressive disorder (O'Reardon et al. 2007). They also demonstrated the following demographic and clinical features:

Table 2–2. Clinical factors to consider when recommending transcranial magnetic stimulation (TMS)

Factor		Additional consideration
Diagnosis	Recurrent depressive illness (unipolar or bipolar)	Current FDA label is for unipolar depression only.
Duration of illness	No defined limitations	Duration <3 years may predict better response.
Level of treatment resistance	At least one trial at or above minimum dose and duration in the current episode	FDA label states any number of treatment failures.
Symptom severity	Moderate to severe	For example, patient has a PHQ-9 score >10.
Age	No defined limitations	Current FDA label is for patients ages 22–70 years.
Sex	No difference in efficacy	
Medical problems	No defined limitations	Patients must be ambulatory and able to cooperate.
Contraindications	No ferromagnetic object within 30 cm of coil	
Precautions	Implanted medical devices	TMS has been safely administered to patients with pacemakers, implantable cardioverter defibrillators, vagus nerve stimulators, and/or deep brain stimulation electrodes.
	Seizure disorder	Optimize anticonvulsant; consider low-frequency TMS.
	Pregnancy/postpartum	TMS has been safely administered to patients who were pregnant or breastfeeding.
	Psychiatric comorbidity	Monitor for emergence of mania or suicidal ideation.

Note. FDA=U.S. Food and Drug Administration; PHQ-9=9-item Patient Health Questionnaire.

Moderate to severe treatment resistance

- Patients experienced between one and four failed research-grade antidepressant medication trials (mean=1.6) in the current episode and received from 1 to as many as 23 trials in total (i.e., adequate and inadequate) to validate the presence of true pharmacological resistance.
- There was no limit to the total number of lifetime treatment attempts.

Moderate to severe symptoms

- Nearly 50% of patients were unemployed because of their depression.
- Nearly 30% of patients were receiving disability payments because of their depression.

Recurrent course of illness

- Over 95% of patients had experienced prior episodes.
- The average age was about 48 years, reflecting a population that was about 10 years older than a first-episode patient population.

These characteristics describe a patient population with a significant degree of treatment resistance. For patients whose depression has not responded to standard first- and second-line treatments, further antidepressant medication treatment would likely involve the use of older medications such as tricyclic antidepressants and monoamine oxidase inhibitors in addition to augmentation strategies such as lithium, thyroid hormone, or second-generation antipsychotics. The risk of discontinuation of antidepressant medication treatment because of side effects increases dramatically, as demonstrated in the STAR*D study, in which the likelihood of discontinuation tripled after one treatment failure and quintupled after three treatment failures (Rush 2007). For such a patient population, electroconvulsive therapy (ECT) would often be the next step, but TMS now offers a well-tolerated alternative for some of these patients (see Chapter 7, "Transcranial Magnetic Stimulation and Other Neuromodulation Therapies").

CLINICAL VIGNETTE

The patient is a 63-year-old woman with a long history of major depression who remained symptomatic despite ongoing treatment. The current episode began 4 years earlier when she moved from the small town where she grew up to a major metropolitan area. At the time of evaluation, she was taking venlafaxine extended-release 150 mg/day, lithium carbonate 600 mg twice daily, and quetiapine 200 mg every night. Previous antidepressant medications in the current episode included once a day dosages of fluoxetine 40 mg, sertraline 150 mg, and citalopram 40 mg. All medication trials lasted at least 8 weeks. Her treatment also included trials of psychotherapy and various augmentation agents.

Her mother committed suicide when the patient was age 9, and the patient's first episode of depression at age 14 involved a suicide attempt by drug overdose. She was hospitalized three times, and a course of ECT when she was in her mid-50s was clinically effective but caused persistent memory deficits. Despite having had brief periods of relative well-being, she never achieved full or sustained remission.

Her score on the 9-item Patient Health Questionnaire (PHQ-9) at the time of evaluation was 26, indicating the presence of severe depression with persistent suicidal thoughts but without specific intent or plan. Her score on the Generalized Anxiety Disorder 7-item scale (GAD-7) was 21, indicating the presence of severe anxiety. She was unable to drive, was housebound, had lost contact with nearly all her friends, and had given up her usual activities. Medical problems included obesity, hyperlipidemia, and chronic obstructive pulmonary disease.

The patient received a total of 36 TMS treatments using 10-Hz, left-sided DLPFC stimulation. Evidence of improvement did not appear until relatively late in her treatment course, but at the conclusion of treatment her PHQ-9 and GAD-7 scores had decreased to zero and her symptoms were in remission. Her response was confirmed by her family and primary psychiatrist, whom she had seen prior to TMS treatment. She continued under the care of her primary psychiatrist and continued taking venlafaxine, but lithium and quetiapine were gradually discontinued. Six months after completing her course of TMS, the patient remained in remission. In addition, she lost 25 pounds, resumed an active social life, was driving again, and returned to her usual interests.

PARTIAL RESPONDERS TO PHARMACOTHERAPY

Patients who achieve a partial response to medication treatment may achieve remission with adjunctive TMS.

CLINICAL VIGNETTE

The patient is a 42-year-old married man who is a small business owner. The current episode of illness began 3 years earlier after the birth of his second child. His wife worked full-time and traveled, and his first child was somewhat "demanding." The patient found weekends increasingly difficult and had given up several hobbies and friendships. He presented for a TMS consultation after reading about it online and completing an online PHQ-9, scoring 12 (moderate).

Prior to his TMS consultation, he shared his concerns and PHQ-9 score with his outpatient psychiatrist, whom he saw every 6 months for prescription refills. His psychiatrist was surprised by the score but also reminded the patient that when he was first diagnosed, his PHQ-9 score was 20. The psychiatrist advised mood monitoring and refilled his prescriptions for duloxetine 90 mg once daily and bupropion extended-release 300 mg once daily.

At his TMS consultation, the patient was diagnosed with major depression, single episode, moderate severity. He received a total of 26 TMS treatments. Within 2 weeks, his PHQ-9 score dropped to 6, and by week 3 he was in remission. TMS was then tapered over the course of 3 weeks. When seen at follow-up 3 months later, he reported that he had reconnected with friends and had started golfing again. However, he complained of sexual side effects, and duloxetine was tapered and discontinued. He remained in remission on bupropion extended-release and later reported that he had resumed sexual relations with his wife.

PATIENTS WITH PSYCHIATRIC COMORBIDITY

Nearly 75% of patients who experience depression will also meet criteria for at least one other mental health disorder, with anxiety (59%) and substance use disorders (24%) being the most common (Kessler et al. 2003). In the naturalistic observational study of acute TMS outcomes in "real-world" patients by Carpenter et al. (2012), 15% of the patients had a comorbid anxiety disorder that did not adversely affect TMS response or remission rates. Patients with long-standing depression often develop maladaptive coping styles and may be misdiagnosed with a personality disorder, especially if treatment does not seem to work. These behaviors may remit when depressive symptoms are effectively treated.

CLINICAL VIGNETTE

The patient is a 42-year-old married woman with a 12-year history of depression. She had a history of superficial wrist cutting and was hospitalized three times. One admission occurred after the police found her on a bridge, where she was contemplating jumping. Her husband is an engineer at a nuclear power plant whose work requires him to be away three times a year for 3 nights in a row. All of her parasuicidal behaviors and hospitalizations occurred when her husband was away. She has been diagnosed with borderline personality disorder and was attending group-based dialectical behavior therapy while taking sertraline 200 mg/day and lithium carbonate 450 mg twice daily. Her PHQ-9 score was 25 and her Montgomery-Åsberg Depression Rating Scale (MADRS) score was 42 at the time of consultation.

After 15 left-sided high-frequency TMS treatments, the patient's PHQ-9 score decreased to 12 and her MADRS score decreased to 20. She began attending her children's after-school sporting events, something she had almost never done previously. After 30 treatments, her PHQ-9 score was 7 and her MADRS score was 12. She remained under the care of her referring psychiatrist and her dialectical behavior therapist, who reported that the patient was making excellent progress in her therapy and was exhibiting a much greater degree of insight than before. When her husband was away, she was able to use newly learned coping skills and did not experience the overwhelming fear of abandonment that she previously had. When she was seen at follow-up 3 months after her treatment course ended, her PHQ-9 score was 6 and her MADRS score was 12.

PATIENTS WITH MEDICAL COMORBIDITY

Major depression rarely occurs in isolation, and medical illnesses such as obesity, cardiovascular disease, and diabetes are common comorbidities. There is no published evidence to date that such a concurrent medical illness has any effect on TMS response, and it is worth repeating that the only contraindication to TMS is the presence of a ferromagnetically sensitive foreign object within 30 cm of the coil placement. There are, however, certain conditions that may require special deliberation when TMS treatment is being considered (see Chapter 3).

Neurological disease is an area of particular interest. Seizure disorders should be optimally controlled. Space-occupying lesions (e.g., tumors) or anatomical abnormalities (e.g., aneurysms) do not necessarily confer a significant risk. Cerebrovascular disease or history of stroke does not preclude a patient from receiving TMS.

Although no laboratory testing is required prior to starting TMS, patients with TRD should be screened for common conditions, such as low levels of vitamin D, low testosterone levels, and hypothyroidism, any of which can cause or exacerbate the core symptoms of depression, such as fatigue, depressed mood, low libido, and cognitive impairment. Obstructive sleep apnea hypopnea syndrome (OSAHS) is another common condition, and it has been estimated that approximately 40% of depressed patients have OSAHS (Harris et al. 2009). Obesity-related hypoventilation with nocturnal hypoxemia is also prevalent. Both conditions are readily diagnosed and treated with continuous positive airway pressure (CPAP) or related techniques, which can sometimes produce rapid and dramatic improvement in depressive symptoms (Schwartz and Karatinos 2007).

CLINICAL VIGNETTE

The patient is a 50-year-old married man with a 12-year history of major depression, which began without a clearly identified precipitant. He saw a news segment about TMS on the local television station and discussed it with his psychiatric nurse practitioner, who agreed it would be reasonable for him to learn more about this option. ECT had already been discussed, but the patient was unwilling to consider it because of concerns about cognitive side effects and the need for repeated general anesthesia.

His QIDS-SR score at the time of evaluation was 22, indicative of a severe depression. He was on disability for 3 years and had abandoned all of his usual hobbies and interests, including woodworking, archery, camping, and playing the guitar. He became sedentary and gained over 50 pounds; developed loud, disruptive snoring that forced him to sleep in a separate bedroom; had no libido and complained of erectile dysfunction; and had not engaged in sexual relations with his wife for over 2 years. He also complained of excessive daytime sleepiness that interfered with his ability to drive for more than 30 minutes.

At the start of treatment, the patient was taking multiple medications, including fluvoxamine 100 mg/day, aripiprazole 30 mg/day, desipramine 100 mg/day, modafinil 200 mg/day, trazodone 75 mg every night, lorazepam 1 mg every night, and alprazolam 0.5 mg three times a day as needed. He had previously experienced five failed trials of other antidepressants, as well as augmentation trials with two second-generation antipsychotics and methylphenidate.

While adhering to this medication regimen, the patient received 36 left-sided high-frequency TMS treatments. His QIDS-SR score on completion was 12. He underwent a sleep study earlier in his course of TMS and began CPAP therapy during his final week of treatment. When he was seen at follow-up 1 month later, his QIDS-SR score was 5, indicating that he was in remission. His sex drive returned along with his ability to achieve and sustain an erection, and because he was no longer snoring, he was again sleeping with his wife. His level of daytime alertness had improved significantly.

He remained under the care of his psychiatric nurse practitioner, but his medication regimen was replaced with transdermal selegiline based on pharmacogenetic test results. When he was seen at follow-up 6 months after his treatment course ended, he was still in remission, had just started a new job, and had resumed all of his previous hobbies.

Preparing the Patient for TMS

Obstacles for patients referred to treatment may include the conviction that they have "tried everything" and will never get better; the belief that they do not deserve to get better; and the expectation that TMS requires a significant commitment of time and effort. All of these matters deserve careful consideration, and it can be helpful to have the patient's spouse, significant other, or a family member present when the treatment is being discussed. This section reviews some of the more common issues that should be addressed with patients and their support network. Clinical information that should be communicated to the TMS center prior to starting treatment is listed in Table 2–3.

Cost is an issue for some patients. Even with widespread insurance coverage for TMS (Tables 2–4 and 2–5), deductibles and copayments may add up to a sizable sum over a course of treatment. Some patients

Table 2–3. Important information to provide when referring a patient for transcranial magnetic stimulation (TMS)

Diagnosis	All psychiatric and medical problems
Current medications	All psychiatric and nonpsychiatric medications, dosages, and indications
Past psychiatric treatment	
Medications	Dates of treatment, maximum dosages, effectiveness, and side effects
Hospitalizations	Locations and dates
Psychotherapy	Providers and dates
Prior neuromodulation	For example, electroconvulsive therapy, vagus nerve stimulation, or prior TMS
Other considerations	For example, overall stability, adherence to treatment, and adequacy of social support network

may be unable or reluctant to incur the expense. They may not recognize the cost of depression itself or the potential financial benefit of being free of depression. It is worth remembering that many depressed patients have difficulty making decisions in general, not just financial decisions. For patients who are truly in need of TMS but lack financial means, third-party medical loans may be appropriate.

Although it is rarely true that a patient has "tried everything," many patients feel that they have. Patients need to understand that depression can always be treated, no matter how long it has persisted or how many prior treatments have failed. Patients should understand that the goal of treatment is not simply to get better but to get well (i.e., to achieve remission). To that end, it can be helpful to review the response and remission rates seen in real-world TMS studies compared with the findings from the STAR*D study. In the real world, most patients who have experienced up to four failed adequate antidepressant medication trials in the current episode will have about a 60% chance of experiencing significant improvement and about a 30% chance of achieving remission with TMS (Carpenter et al. 2012). In a recent open-label trial, patients showed a 60% remission rate after receiving 6 weeks of TMS monotherapy (Philip et al. 2016). Such statistics should be stated in a clear and matter-of-fact manner, in much the same way that a surgeon might explain the relative success rates of a given procedure. Patients must also understand, however, that depression is a chronic and recurrent condition and that even

---

Table 2–4. Private insurance coverage policies for transcranial magnetic stimulation (TMS) therapy

---

General	All major insurance companies have a positive TMS coverage policy.
	Payers vary as to who is or is not covered.
	Some TMS centers do not accept insurance and are not in network for any payers, whereas other TMS centers are in network with select payers.
	Coverage policies change, and patients or providers can access policies by calling the insurance company. Some payers post their policies on the Web.
Diagnosis	All payers require a primary diagnosis of major depressive disorder, recurrent or single episode, of moderate or severe degree. Some payers limit coverage to severe cases.
	All payers require a validated rating of the depression symptoms (e.g., PHQ-9, QIDS).
Age	All payers cover "adult patients"; however, some payers define adult patients in their policies as those ages 22–68, whereas other payers cover patients age 18 years and older.
Treatment resistance	Coverage policies vary on the requirements for number of antidepressants tried and/or psychotherapy.
	Some policies, particularly the commercial plans for federal employees, cover TMS after one failed antidepressant attempt.
	Most policies cover patients once they have tried four or more antidepressants and undergone a trial of psychotherapy in the current episode of depression.
	Most plans require proper documentation of start and stop dates and dosing of treatments tried. These data are submitted for payer review by TMS centers that take insurance to obtain insurance approval for the procedure.
Comorbidity	Some plans limit coverage if the patient has a history of posttraumatic stress disorder, an anxiety diagnosis, or a history of substance abuse.
	Some plans exclude patients who have a history of seizure, who have epilepsy, or who are pregnant.
TMS system	All payers require TMS centers to use TMS systems that have been cleared for use by the U.S. Food and Drug Administration.

Note. PHQ-9=9-item Patient Health Questionnaire; QIDS=Quick Inventory of Depressive Symptomatology.

Table 2–5. Government coverage policies for transcranial magnetic stimulation (TMS) therapy

Medicare	TMS coverage is determined by each Medicare administrative contractor (MAC).
	All MACs cover TMS therapy for adult patients with major depressive disorder.
	Specifics of coverage can be found on the Web as local coverage determinations.
	Coverage criteria vary by MAC or region of the country.
	Coverage criteria by commercial Medicare programs often default to the commercial carrier's coverage criteria.
Medicaid	Coverage is not widely available for Medicaid members.
	Coverage is usually determined by the Medicaid contractor.
VA Medical Centers/ TRICARE	Coverage varies by regions for the VA Medical Centers.
	TRICARE has a positive TMS policy for adults with major depression. Coverage specifics are determined regionally by contractors.

Note. TRICARE=health care program for uniformed service members and their families; VA=Veterans Administration.

with full remission, they will need to continue treatment, usually in the form of antidepressant medication, to sustain improvement (see Chapter 6, "Managing Patients After Transcranial Magnetic Stimulation").

Patients often incorrectly assume that TMS is simply a less noxious form of ECT. It is important for patients to understand how TMS differs from ECT, particularly with respect to the avoidance of seizures and resulting lack of cognitive side effects with TMS (see Chapter 7). Many patients have only a rudimentary understanding of electromagnetism and a limited understanding of brain physiology and the pathophysiology of depression. A plainspoken, nontechnical explanation of the mechanism of action of TMS can be very reassuring and provides important information a patient requires to be able to provide informed consent (see Chapter 3).

All patients who receive TMS have previously taken antidepressant medications and understand that they do not work immediately. Nevertheless, many patients will expect TMS to produce immediate results and may become frustrated and anxious when this does not happen. It is important for patients to understand that improvement typically takes several weeks and that not all symptoms of depression improve at the same rate. This foreknowledge helps patients stay engaged with treatment. It is especially important for patients to understand that "vegetative" symptoms such as sleep, appetite, and energy level typically improve before the subjective symptoms of sadness, emptiness, and despair. Family members or others who know the patient well may notice subtle signs of improvement before the patient does.

Patients may be concerned about the time commitment required to complete a course of TMS, as well as having to take time off from work to attend daily sessions (20–45 minutes/session for 5 days/week for potentially 4–6 weeks or longer). Although some patients may choose to take a medical leave of absence or request time off under the aegis of the Family Medical Leave Act, this is rarely a major problem. Patients can be reassured that because anesthesia and sedation are not required, TMS generally involves no other disruption of their daily routine than the session time required.

Table 2–6 summarizes information that needs to be discussed with patients as they consider whether to undergo TMS treatment.

Conclusion

Characterizing the ideal patient for TMS requires development of more precise methods of defining depression. In response to this dilemma, the National Institute of Mental Health is sponsoring development of research diagnostic criteria that promote the use of biological, neurophysiological, and clinical factors to parse out subgroups of individuals presenting with syndromic depression. The ultimate goal is to provide more specific and therefore more effective treatments. Such efforts represent an important step in the desired direction; however, ongoing work is needed. In the meantime, it is critical to utilize all presently available resources to maximize the chances of alleviating patients' suffering. Although it is still in a phase of ongoing refinement, TMS represents an increasingly important option for treatment-resistant depression.

Table 2–6. Important clinical issues to discuss when explaining transcranial magnetic stimulation (TMS) to patients

---

Depression is a brain disease, not a sign of weakness or failure.

Depression can always be treated regardless of duration, severity, or level of treatment resistance.

TMS is effective in treatment-resistant depression.

TMS uses a special device to stimulate the brain using magnetic resonance imaging–strength magnetic fields.

TMS stimulates a certain part of the brain that is underactive in depression, restoring it to normal function.

TMS is not like electroconvulsive therapy because it does not require the induction of a seizure and it does not cause cognitive side effects.

TMS usually takes 4–6 weeks to produce maximum benefit.

Although most patients experience significant improvement with TMS, the treatment does not work for everyone.

TMS is not a cure, and ongoing treatment is usually necessary to prevent depression from returning.

KEY CLINICAL POINTS

- Depression is a major public health problem and a leading cause of disability worldwide.
- Most patients do not receive adequate treatment for depression, and remission is hard to achieve.
- Up to 30% of patients develop treatment-resistant depression, defined in this chapter as failure to achieve remission after two antidepressant treatment courses of adequate dose and duration.
- TMS is not a treatment of last resort.
- Medical or psychiatric comorbidity is not a contraindication to TMS.
- The only contraindication to TMS is the presence of ferromagnetically sensitive material within 30 cm of the TMS coil.
- Private insurance and Medicare cover TMS therapy for adult patients with major depression who have not responded to or tolerated one or more antidepressant medications.

- The majority of patients who receive TMS experience clinical improvement, and many achieve remission.

- TMS should be viewed as one component of a comprehensive plan of care.

References

Carpenter LL, Janicak PG, Aaronson ST, et al: Transcranial magnetic stimulation (TMS) for major depression: a multisite, naturalistic, observational study of acute treatment outcomes in clinical practice. Depress Anxiety 29(7):587–596, 2012 22689344

Goldman LS, Nielsen NH, Champion HC; Council on Scientific Affairs, American Medical Association: Awareness, diagnosis, and treatment of depression. J Gen Intern Med 14(9):569–580, 1999 10491249

Harris M, Glozier N, Ratnavadivel R, et al: Obstructive sleep apnea and depression. Sleep Med Rev 13(6):437–444, 2009 19596599

Katon W, Von Korff M, Lin E, et al: Adequacy and duration of antidepressant treatment in primary care. Med Care 30(1):67–76, 1992 1729588

Kessler RC, Berglund P, Demler O, et al; National Comorbidity Survey Replication: The epidemiology of major depressive disorder: results from the National Comorbidity Survey Replication (NCS-R). JAMA 289(23):3095–3105, 2003 12813115

Lisanby SH, Husain MM, Rosenquist PB, et al: Daily left prefrontal repetitive transcranial magnetic stimulation in the acute treatment of major depression: clinical predictors of outcome in a multisite, randomized controlled clinical trial. Neuropsychopharmacology 34(2):522–534, 2009 18704101

O'Reardon JP, Solvason HB, Janicak PG, et al: Efficacy and safety of transcranial magnetic stimulation in the acute treatment of major depression: a multisite randomized controlled trial. Biol Psychiatry 62(11):1208–1216, 2007 17573044

Philip NS, Dunner DL, Dowd SM, et al: Can medication free, treatment-resistant, depressed patients who initially respond to TMS be maintained off medications? A prospective, 12-month multisite randomized pilot study. Brain Stimul 9(2):251–257, 2016 26708778

Pratt LA, Brody DJ: Depression in the U.S. Household Population, 2009–2012. NCHS Data Brief, No 172. Hyattsville, MD, National Center for Health Statistics, 2014

Rush AJ: STAR*D: what have we learned? Am J Psychiatry 164(2):201–214, 2007 17267779

Schwartz DJ, Karatinos G: For individuals with obstructive sleep apnea, institution of CPAP therapy is associated with an amelioration of symptoms of depression which is sustained long term. J Clin Sleep Med 3(6):631–635, 2007 17993046

Substance Abuse and Mental Health Services Administration: Key suBstance Use and Mental Health Indicators in the United States: Results From the 2015 National Survey on Drug Use and Health (HHS Publ No SMA 16-4984, NSDUH Series H-51). September 2016. Available at: https://www.samhsa.gov/data/sites/default/files/NSDUH-FFR1-2015/NSDUH-FFR1-2015/NSDUH-FFR1-2015.pdf. Accessed April 3, 2017.

Warden D, Rush AJ, Trivedi MH, et al: The STAR*D project results: a comprehensive review of findings. Curr Psychiatry Rep 9(6):449–459, 2007 18221624

Risk Management Issues in Transcranial Magnetic Stimulation for Treatment of Major Depression

Philip G. Janicak, M.D.

A determination about the overall effectiveness of any therapy should take into account the therapy's efficacy, safety, and tolerability and a patient's willingness to accept and adhere to it. In this chapter, I review the safety and tolerability of repetitive transcranial magnetic stimulation (TMS), focusing on its use for the treatment of depression. In these respects, TMS compares favorably with alternative therapies for major depression, including medications and other neuromodulation approaches such as electroconvulsive therapy (ECT) and vagus nerve stimulation.

This low-risk profile is supported by results from numerous preclinical and clinical studies, as well as increasing practical experience since the first TMS device was cleared by the U.S. Food and Drug Administration (FDA) for treatment of depression in 2008 (Rossi et al. 2009). One caveat in interpreting data generated from controlled clinical trials is that the researchers have typically used TMS as a monotherapy. By contrast, clinicians typically use TMS as an adjunct to various medications, potentially altering the risk of certain adverse events (AEs). Overall, TMS has a very favorable safety and tolerability profile when compared with medications (e.g., TMS has minimal systemic effects) and other neuromodulation therapies (e.g., TMS is noninvasive and nonconvulsive). As a result, the retention rates in clinical trials were much better than with standard therapies, further improving the chances of a favorable outcome (see Chapter 4, "Combining Pharmacotherapy With Transcranial Magnetic Stimulation in the Treatment of Major Depression").

This chapter begins with a description of the initial evaluation process, which should include an appropriate informed consent to facilitate the patient's decision making regarding TMS. Next, the most common AEs associated with TMS; the uncommon but more serious potential for an inadvertent seizure; specific risks across the life cycle (i.e., TMS during the perinatal period, in children and adolescents, in the elderly); other potential safety and tolerability issues (e.g., auditory changes, potential for tissue injury, cognitive effects); and alternative approaches are discussed.

TMS Evaluation Process

The TMS evaluation process begins with the determination of a patient's eligibility for TMS. Two crucial components of this process are confirming diagnostic criteria and assessing the patient's ability to understand and accept the risk/benefit aspects of TMS.

To ensure informed consent after the diagnostic review, adequate time is needed for the professional to describe the components of a TMS device; the motor threshold (MT) determination procedure; a typical treatment session; a typical treatment course; the chances of response and remission; the most common AEs; the potential for a seizure; and other possible risks specific to an individual's circumstances (e.g., medication regimen, medical history).

To minimize the potential risks associated with TMS, its prescription should be written by a licensed physician or other professional (e.g., an advanced practice nurse) with prescriptive authority. At a minimum, the treating professional and staff should be adequately trained and certified by the TMS device manufacturer. Recent professional consensus

Table 3–1. Transcranial magnetic stimulation: guidelines for safe administration

Guideline	Action
Adequate risk/benefit assessment	Screen for contraindications/warnings
Informed consent	Discuss thoroughly what to expect
No routine labs or imaging required unless indicated	NA
Prescription for TMS	Obtain written prescription from licensed physician or another professional with prescriptive authority

guidelines also recommend initial peer-to-peer direct supervision and ongoing, documented educational experiences (e.g., continuing medical education [CME] programs) to maintain and enhance competency (Perera et al. 2016).

Table 3–1 summarizes the guidelines for safe administration of TMS. These include assessing the risk-benefit ratio for TMS in each patient; securing informed consent; considering the need for laboratory assessments as dictated by a patient's history (e.g., thyroid function tests, sleep study); and obtaining a specific prescription for the TMS procedure.

Common Adverse Events

The most common AEs associated with TMS include *application site discomfort* (e.g., scalp pain under the area where the coil is placed) and *events due to direct stimulation of neural tissue*. Some common examples of the latter events include trigeminal nerve–related pain, contraction of muscles around the eye, lachrymation, and toothaches, all of which occur primarily during delivery of the stimulation train. Tension-like *headaches* may also occur after a treatment session because of contraction of muscle tissue near the coil (Janicak et al. 2008). See Table 3–2.

Although a majority of patients experience these events, usually they are tolerable and/or progressively subside in intensity during the treatment course because of rapid accommodation and the ability of the technician to alter various treatment parameters (usually temporarily) or to change coil positioning to enhance comfort. As a result, discontinuation due to AEs associated with TMS therapy is relatively low (e.g., ~5% in sham-controlled trials).

Table 3–2. Adverse events associated with two transcranial magnetic stimulation (TMS) systems: results from three studies

	NeuroStar TMS Therapy System	**Brainsway Deep TMS System**
Description	Biphasic figure eight with ferromagnetic core	H coil with air core, air cooling
Study participants	$N=491$ (studies 1 and 2)	$N=181$
FDA clearance	2008	2013
Deaths/suicides or suicide attempts	Study 1: 1 apparent suicidal gesture (sham patient)	None
Suicide ideation	Study 1: worsening suicidality (1 active patient; 10 sham patients)	Not reported
Common adverse events	Headache and application site pain	Headache and application site pain
		15% of the ITT sample were excluded because they were treated at a lower intensity because of presumed intolerability at full intensity
Significant adverse events	Study 1: 16 SAEs (9 active patients; 7 sham patients; primarily symptom worsening)	8 SAEs (4 sham patients; 3 active patients; 1 patient prior to randomization)
	Study 2: 3 SAEs (1 patient prior to randomization; 1 active patient with syncope; 1 sham patient with paranoia)	1 SAE considered device related (i.e., a seizure in an active patient)
Cognition	No effects	No effects
Discontinuation rate due to adverse events	~5%	1%
References	Study 1: Janicak et al. 2008 Study 2: George et al. 2010	Levkovitz et al. 2015

Note. FDA=U.S. Food and Drug Administration; ITT=intent-to-treat; SAE=significant adverse event.

Specific strategies to improve tolerability of the TMS procedure include 1) rotating the coil angle, 2) moving the coil slightly more anteriorly or laterally, 3) temporarily lowering the stimulus intensity, and 4) applying lidocaine anesthetic cream to the skin under the coil. Headaches are usually controlled by over-the-counter analgesics, which are taken at the onset of symptoms or before a treatment session to prevent the repeated occurrence of headaches. Occasionally, for patients who continue to experience intolerable AEs, switching to a low-frequency (i.e., 1 Hz or less) stimulation protocol over the right dorsolateral prefrontal cortex (DLPFC) has led to a successfully completed course of TMS (Brunelin et al. 2014).

CLINICAL VIGNETTE

The patient is a 33-year-old man experiencing his second episode of major depression. During his previous episode, at age 22, he had difficulty tolerating several trials of medication, which contributed to a worsening of his symptoms, particularly more severe suicidality. He then had a course of ECT, to which he responded, but he also experienced significant memory loss that took several months to clear. He now requests a trial of TMS in the hope that it will resolve this episode without his having to undergo poorly tolerated medication trials or another course of ECT and the resultant memory problems. Of note, the patient is presently experiencing only passive suicidality and has no psychotic symptoms. He initiates a course of TMS but experiences substantial application site pain, which is ameliorated with a reduction in his MT level to 100%. Over the next five sessions, the level is gradually increased as tolerated to the targeted 120% of MT. After a successful course of acute TMS, based on improvement in his scores on the 9-item Patient Health Questionnaire (PHQ-9), the patient's clinician prescribes maintenance cognitive-behavioral therapy as well as TMS sessions at a frequency determined by a gradual reduction protocol over several weeks.

Seizure Risk With TMS

Although seizure risk is the most serious potential TMS-related AE, seizures are uncommon. The most recent data indicate an estimated risk of less than 0.1% over an entire treatment course (typically 20–30 sessions) (Dobek et al. 2015).

Of note, all documented TMS-induced seizures have occurred during treatment sessions. The risk of seizures during TMS compares favorably with risks from various psychotropic medications (e.g., antipsychotics, tricyclic antidepressants, bupropion) used to treat depression. Paradoxically, a recent systematic review indicates that *TMS may suppress* episodes in patients with epilepsy (Pereira et al. 2016). Although a patient's history of seizures or a seizure disorder does not pose an absolute contraindication to TMS, this issue should be carefully explored with the patient and appropriately addressed. Safeguards may include discontinuation of medications, which can lower the seizure threshold; adjustment in anticonvulsant medications to ensure adequate control; and consultation with a neurologist.

Minimizing the risk of seizures begins with a careful assessment of factors that can increase seizure potential. These include a history of prior head injuries, stroke, brain lesions (e.g., vascular, traumatic, infectious), and/or seizure events; recent sleep deprivation; and the use of medications, alcohol, or other substances that may lower the seizure threshold. Administering TMS treatments within the recommended parameters (e.g., frequency, intensity, coil location, train duration, intertrain interval) is a crucial step in minimizing seizure risk. Because adhering to the suggested parameters may not always be possible, when parameters go beyond standard settings, patients should be informed of a potentially higher risk for a seizure.

After the initial assessment and appropriate modification of risk factors, it is important that staff frequently re-inquire about any changes in the patient's status during the course of treatment. A corollary to such monitoring is the need for ongoing communication with the patient's support system and primary treatment team. Table 3–3 includes a list of issues to be assessed prior to initiating TMS.

If confronted with a possible event, the treatment staff should clarify whether it is a vasovagal syncope, which may be more common than and can mimic some aspects of a seizure. Because of the possibilities of seizures and syncopal events, it is important that a licensed provider always be available on site for consultation when treatments are being provided. Furthermore, first-response training to manage a seizure episode is mandatory for all treating staff. Additionally, it is critical that the technician who typically administers the treatments has the appropriate background and training and is present throughout a session to monitor the patient. Although technicians' backgrounds may vary, many are medically trained (e.g., registered nurses, licensed practical nurses, emergency medical technicians) and adept in techniques to maintain airway, breathing, and circulation. Because some sites use technicians with no formal credentials or licensure, however, additional training may be necessary.

Reports of TMS-related seizure events indicate that a relatively short time passes before spontaneous resolution (e.g., ~60 seconds) with no residual neurological or medical sequelae. Therefore, there is some debate about the need for on-site emergency equipment (e.g., oxygen, suction,

Table 3–3. Issues to address prior to transcranial magnetic stimulation (TMS)

Patient's history

  Epilepsy or seizure

  Fainting spell(s) or syncope

  Head trauma, concussion, or loss of consciousness

  Hearing problems, ringing in the ears

  Prior TMS treatment and any associated problems

  Prior magnetic resonance imaging and any associated problems

Patient's current conditions

  Presence and type of metal substance in the brain, skull, or elsewhere in the body

  Presence of implanted device (e.g., cochlear implant, direct brain stimulation device, vagus nerve stimulation device)

  Presence of cardiac pacemaker or intracardiac lines

  Presence of medication infusion device

  Current medications

  Pregnancy

Source.   Adapted from Rossi et al. 2011.

intravenous medications). Regardless, the most important protective steps to prevent complications when a syncopal or seizure event occurs include stopping the TMS session; positioning the chair and the patient to prevent falls, asphyxiation, and aspiration; and calling for emergency personnel. Venous access and anticonvulsants may also be available but are not typically needed.

Finally, all TMS centers should have an approved seizure policy and procedure that has been thoroughly reviewed by treating personnel and is kept in a readily accessible location.

CLINICAL VIGNETTE

The patient is a 45-year-old woman with a 20-year history of recurrent major depression. Her present episode has lasted 2 years and, unlike her previous episodes, has not adequately responded to standard medication and cognitive-behavioral therapy trials. She has no psychotic symptoms and only passive thoughts of suicide with no intent or plan. A course of TMS is deemed appropriate, but her present medication regimen includes nortriptyline (150 mg/day) plus aripiprazole (5 mg/day) for augmentation, and the patient has increased her daily alcohol use to manage her mood symptoms and medication-related AEs. Her medications, as well as her increased alcohol consumption and possible related withdrawal phenomena, can lower the seizure threshold. Because the patient reports anxiety/akathisia but no benefit from aripiprazole, the medication is stopped for 2 weeks prior to assessment of the patient's MT. She is also started on lorazepam (1 mg twice daily) and naltrexone (50 mg/day) to control her anxiety/akathisia, to counteract any symptoms associated with her agreed-on cessation of alcohol, and to decrease cravings. While continuing her nortriptyline, lorazepam, and naltrexone, the patient successfully completes her course of TMS without incident.

TMS Risks Across the Life Cycle

PERINATAL PERIOD

The management of depression during pregnancy raises critical issues about how to balance the negative impact to the fetus from an inadequately controlled maternal mood disorder and related symptoms versus the potential deleterious effects of medications. Although ECT remains a viable treatment alternative, especially for more severe life-threatening episodes, it carries significant risks (e.g., need for repeated anesthetic exposures and maternal seizure inductions, fetal heart rate changes, maternal cognitive AEs). These risks have led to consideration of TMS as a possible treatment option. Thus far, however, TMS has only been considered in case reports and open-label pilot studies using right-sided low-frequency treatments to limit seizure risk (Kim et al. 2015). Results of an ongoing sham-controlled trial of TMS should provide better information about the treatment's clinical benefit in this population and clarify whether there are any systemic effects that may negatively impact the fetus (see Chapter 8, "Transcranial Magnetic Stimulation for the Treatment of Other Mood Disorders").

CHILDHOOD AND ADOLESCENCE

Presently, limited data are available on the safety and tolerability of repetitive TMS in younger age groups. According to a review involving more than 513 children and adolescents (ages 2.5–17.8 years) with various neurological and psychiatric disorders, this population generally experienced only mild and transient TMS-related AEs, including headaches, 11.5%; scalp discomfort, 2.5%; twitching, 1.2%; mood changes, 1.2%; fatigue, 0.9%; and tinnitus, 0.6% (Krishnan et al. 2015). A subsequent report noted a seizure event in a 17-year-old depressed girl who was not taking any medications and who had no contributory medical, neurological, or substance use history (Cullen et al. 2016). While participating in a trial with deep TMS (a technique described in section "Alternative Approaches" below), the patient experienced a tonic-clonic seizure during her eighth treatment session; the seizure resolved in 90 seconds with no sequelae or need for anticonvulsant medications. At 6-month follow-up, she was reported to be doing well. The authors suggest that additional precautions and further dose-finding studies with deep TMS are needed for this age group (see Chapter 8).

OLDER AGE

Ironically, older adults are usually excluded from clinical trials, but they represent a substantial proportion of individuals with treatment-resistant depression (TRD). Although ECT is frequently administered to this population, associated AEs (particularly cognitive) are often a concern for staff, patients, and families.

For older adults, TMS is considered a possible alternative given its apparent absence of adverse cognitive effects (see section "Other Potential Risk Issues" below), lower cost, and evidence of greater patient preference (Magnezi et al. 2016). Early in the clinical development of TMS, however, concerns about its effectiveness were raised because of the increased coil-to-cortex distance in the elderly due to age-related brain atrophy. More recently, the standard use of higher stimulation levels (e.g., 120% of MT) appears to address this issue; a meta-analysis found that older age did not predict lack of benefit and higher stimulation levels were well tolerated (Berlim et al. 2014). Given the need for more effective and more tolerable treatments for this age group, definitive studies are needed to confirm the usefulness of TMS (Blumberger et al. 2015) (see Chapter 8).

Other Potential Risk Issues

PSYCHIATRIC COMPLICATIONS ASSOCIATED WITH TMS

Both *psychosis* (rarely) and *mania* (more commonly) are reported as treatment-emergent AEs with TMS, but causality is not clearly established and event rates appear to be within the expectable natural ranges. If TMS is used off-label for bipolar depression, monitoring for emerging hypomania/mania is critical. Also, if a mood switch occurs, stopping antidepressant medications, adding mood stabilizers, reducing TMS session frequency, or stopping TMS may be appropriate steps. Known bipolar patients should also be taking adequate mood-stabilizing medication(s) prior to starting TMS (Xia et al. 2008) (see discussion of TMS treatment of bipolar depression in Chapter 8).

Reassuringly, evidence for worsening of *suicidality* with active TMS was absent in the largest sham-controlled trial to date (e.g., Janicak et al. 2008). In addition, induction of psychosis and suicidality have not been reported in nondepressed subjects receiving TMS. Despite these encouraging data, given that the more highly suicidal patients were excluded from the major studies, caution is advised and ongoing monitoring for such emergent symptoms is important. Therefore, clinicians should choose the most appropriate venue to first stabilize patients who are at higher suicide risk, be aware that TMS can take 4–6 weeks to achieve an adequate antidepressant effect, and arrange for patients receiving TMS as outpatients to be in a setting with proper support and monitoring. Alternatively, TMS can be administered in an inpatient setting that provides the appropriate level of care.

AUDITORY CHANGES

Because TMS devices can generate noise levels beyond 140 decibels and the coil is located close to a patient's ear, the use of disposable earplugs is recommended for both the patient and the treatment technician. In the three largest controlled trials of TMS for depression, each of which used earplugs, there was no evidence of auditory compromise (George et al. 2010; Levkovitz et al. 2015; O'Reardon et al. 2007). Despite these data, there are concerns that higher stimulation intensities, with their associated increases in noise levels, may still pose problems in young children and produce transient hearing disturbances in adequately protected adults (Rossi et al. 2009; Tringali et al. 2012).

COGNITIVE EFFECTS

In contrast to ECT and certain medications for depression, low-frequency repetitive TMS over the right DLPFC does not appear to cause any cognitive issues in various patient populations, including patients with mood disorders (Lage et al. 2016). Furthermore, in the largest ($N=301$) sham-controlled trial of high-frequency repetitive TMS over the left DLPFC for treatment of major depression, Janicak et al. (2008) found no changes in global cognitive function, short-term and delayed recall, or retrieval of long-term autobiographical memory. Also, Schulze et al. (2016) reported that TMS applied over the medial prefrontal cortex in 21 patients with TRD did not produce any detectable cognitive AEs. Finally, in a trial of sequential bilateral TMS in 63 patients with TRD, Galletly et al. (2016) found no significant cognitive impairment as assessed by a robust battery of computerized cognitive tests. As noted in the section "TMS Risks Across the Life Cycle," TMS may be particularly helpful in vulnerable populations such as the elderly. Indeed, preliminary data indicate a possible procognitive effect in patients with mild to moderate Alzheimer's dementia treated with high-frequency TMS over both the left and right DLPFCs (Ahmed et al. 2012).

CELLULAR CHANGES

There is no clear evidence of nervous system tissue damage associated with TMS as presently used to treat depression (Janicak et al. 2008). The intermittent gradient field produced by TMS is comparable to that used in magnetic resonance imaging (MRI) in terms of field peak intensity and switching times. Thus, similar levels of current density are induced in conductive tissue, resulting in negligible heating and no evidence of cellular changes or mutagenesis. Also, total pulsed field exposure is orders of magnitude less with TMS than in a standard MRI session.

METALLIC OBJECTS, IMPLANTED PHYSIOLOGICALLY CONTROLLED ELECTRODES, AND RELATED DEVICES

Any *ferromagnetic material, internal pulse generators,* or *medication pumps within 30 cm* of the coil placement constitute contraindications to TMS, as do *cochlear implants.* These objects present potential risks during TMS primarily due to potential heating effects from the magnetic field and damage to the internal circuitry of nearby implanted devices. *Dental implants* made with magnetically sensitive materials and located on the side of stimulation are also contraindications. Exceptions include dental hardware and titanium metals that have low conductivity and therefore pose little risk for damage to surrounding tissues (Rossi et al. 2009). Before a treatment session, anything worn on the head or neck that has conductive potential (e.g., jewelry, glasses) should be removed.

Cardiac pacemakers, vagus nerve stimulation systems, spinal cord stimulators, and brain implants (e.g., aneurysm clips) pose a relative contraindication for TMS due to potential tissue injury related to mechanical movement induced by the rapidly alternating magnetic fields with TMS. Conventional TMS output, however, appears to remain below that necessary to cause tissue damage, and most device components are usually beyond the TMS-generated electromagnetic field (Golestanirad et al. 2012). Therefore, TMS may still be administered but with consideration given to the location of these implants relative to the coil and the need for appropriate precautions (e.g., reduced transcranial magnetic stimulus intensity). In these cases, more specific consent procedures addressing any of these issues and consultation with a specialist are recommended.

Additionally, stimulation electrodes as in deep brain stimulation should be considered a contraindication for TMS until further safety studies can be conducted.

Alternative Approaches

Although low-frequency right DLPFC and low-frequency synchronized TMS (not presently available for clinical use) may reduce risks such as seizures, their efficacy compared with left-sided high-frequency TMS is not clearly established (Leuchter et al. 2015). In contrast, other stimulation protocols such as *deep TMS* and *theta burst stimulation* (TBS) theoretically pose additional risks.

Deep TMS, which received FDA clearance in 2013, uses alternative coil technology and configurations (e.g., helmet-like H coil) to achieve more direct stimulation of relevant structures (e.g., cingulate gyrus) (Levkovitz et al. 2015). Increased depth of stimulation, however, comes at the cost of higher frequencies (e.g., 18 Hz) and less focality, which possibly increase seizure risk, especially in more vulnerable populations such as adolescents (Bersani et al. 2013; Cullen et al. 2016).

TBS is a patterned form of magnetic pulse delivery that intersperses higher (e.g., 50 Hz) and lower frequencies within the same stimulus train (Janicak et al. 2016). Such an approach could significantly reduce administration time, reduce costs, and increase patient acceptability. Although such higher frequencies could theoretically increase seizure risk, the existing results in adults and youth under age 18 years have not borne this out. Although TBS is being used off-label in clinical practice, additional studies are needed, and therefore, appropriate caution is suggested (Hong et al. 2015; Oberman et al. 2011).

Conclusion

Repetitive TMS, per the guidelines approved by the FDA, is a remarkably safe and well-tolerated therapy. TMS results in minimal systemic effects and lacks adverse interactions compared with medication. Also, there is no need to induce a seizure and the associated cognitive adverse events as occur with electroconvulsive therapy, and there is no need for an invasive surgical procedure as with vagus nerve stimulation. TMS-related adverse events appear to be comparable whether TMS is used as a monotherapy or in combination with medications or other neuromodulation approaches. Although data in special populations and with longer-term exposure are less extensive, it is reassuring that the safety and tolerability profile for TMS seems to persist in such uses (Dunner et al. 2014; Janicak et al. 2010). Proper training of qualified personnel is paramount to ensure this high benefit-to-risk ratio. Ongoing efforts to enhance the efficacy of TMS for depression and to expand its indications must in part be guided by the need to maintain the present favorable safety and tolerability profile. Continuing research promises to clarify and hopefully enhance TMS's efficacy, safety, and tolerability in treating patients with depression, as well as other populations (see Chapters 8, "Transcranial Magnetic Stimulation for the Treatment of Other Mood Disorders," and 9, "Transcranial Magnetic Stimulation for Disorders Other Than Depression").

KEY CLINICAL POINTS

- Referring psychiatrists can assure patients that TMS is a very safe and well-tolerated therapy.

- TMS possesses a relatively high benefit-to-risk ratio compared with other biological therapies for depression, with minimal systemic effects (e.g., weight gain, sexual dysfunction); no cognitive problems; and only one clear contraindication (i.e., ferrometallic material, internal pulse generators, and medication pumps within 30 cm of the coil placement).

- No anesthesia is required, and patients remain completely independent during all aspects of the treatment process (e.g., no driving restrictions).

- The most common adverse events associated with TMS (e.g., application site discomfort, muscle tension–related headaches) are generally tolerable, are readily managed, and rarely lead to discontinuation of treatment.

- Although seizure risk is very low and most contributory factors can be anticipated and controlled, seizure represents the most serious TMS-related adverse event.

- Ongoing communication with a patient's social system, primary psychiatrist, and other treatment professionals serves as an invaluable source of collateral information, helping to avoid unnecessary changes in concomitant therapies, which may increase the risks and/or undermine the benefits of TMS.

References

Ahmed MA, Darwish ES, Khedr EM, et al: Effects of low versus high frequencies of repetitive transcranial magnetic stimulation on cognitive function and cortical excitability in Alzheimer's dementia. J Neurol 259(1):83–92, 2012 21671144

Berlim MT, van den Eynde F, Tovar-Perdomo S, et al: Response, remission and drop-out rates following high-frequency repetitive transcranial magnetic stimulation (rTMS) for treating major depression: a systematic review and meta-analysis of randomized, double-blind and sham-controlled trials. Psychol Med 44(2):225–239, 2014 23507264

Bersani FS, Minichino A, Enticott PG, et al: Deep transcranial magnetic stimulation as a treatment for psychiatric disorders: a comprehensive review. Eur Psychiatry 28(1):30–39, 2013 22559998

Blumberger DM, Hsu JH, Daskalakis ZJ: A review of brain stimulation treatments for late-life depression. Curr Treat Options Psychiatry 2(4):413–421, 2015 27398288

Brunelin J, Jalenques I, Trojak B, et al; STEP Group: The efficacy and safety of low frequency repetitive transcranial magnetic stimulation for treatment-resistant depression: the results from a large multicenter French RCT. Brain Stimul 7(6):855–863, 2014 25192980

Cullen KR, Jasberg S, Nelson B, et al: Seizure induced by deep transcranial magnetic stimulation in an adolescent with depression. J Child Adolesc Psychopharmacol 26(7):637–641, 2016 27447245

Dobek CE, Bumberger DM, Downar J, Daskalakis ZJ, et al: Risk of seizures in transcranial magnetic stimulation: a clinical review to inform consent process focused on bupropion. Neuropsychiatr Dis Treat 11:2975–2987, 2015 26664122

Dunner DL, Aaronson ST, Sackeim HA, et al: A multisite, naturalistic, observational study of transcranial magnetic stimulation for patients with pharmacoresistant major depressive disorder: durability of benefit over a 1-year follow-up period. J Clin Psychiatry 75(12):1394–1401, 2014 25271871

Galletly C, Gill S, Rigby A, et al: Assessing the effects of repetitive transcranial magnetic stimulation on cognition in major depressive disorder using computerized cognitive testing. J ECT 32(3):169–173, 2016 26934275

George MS, Lisanby SH, Avery D, et al: Daily left prefrontal transcranial magnetic stimulation therapy for major depressive disorder: a sham-controlled randomized trial. Arch Gen Psychiatry 67(5):507–516, 2010 20439832

Golestanirad L, Rouhani H, Elahi B, et al: Combined use of transcranial magnetic stimulation and metal electrode implants: a theoretical assessment of safety considerations. Phys Med Biol 57(23):7813–7827, 2012 23135209

Hong YH, Wu SW, Pedapati EV, et al: Safety and tolerability of theta burst stimulation vs. single and paired pulse transcranial magnetic stimulation: a comparative study of 165 pediatric subjects. Front Hum Neurosci 9:29, 2015 25698958

Janicak PG, O'Reardon JP, Sampson SM, et al: Transcranial magnetic stimulation in the treatment of major depressive disorder: a comprehensive summary of safety experience from acute exposure, extended exposure, and during reintroduction treatment. J Clin Psychiatry 69(2):222–232, 2008 18232722

Janicak PG, Nahas Z, Lisanby SH, et al: Durability of clinical benefit with transcranial magnetic stimulation (TMS) in the treatment of pharmacoresistant major depression: assessment of relapse during a 6-month, multisite, open-label study. Brain Stimulat 3(4):187–199, 2010 20965447

Janicak PG, Sackett V, Kudrna K, et al: Advances in transcranial magnetic stimulation for managing major depressive disorders. Curr Psychiatr 15(6):49–56, 2016

Kim DR, Snell JL, Ewing GC, et al: Neuromodulation and antenatal depression: a review. Neuropsychiatr Dis Treat 11:975–982, 2015 25897234

Krishnan C, Santos L, Peterson MD, et al: Safety of noninvasive brain stimulation in children and adolescents. Brain Stimulat 8(1):76–87, 2015 25499471

Lage C, Wiles K, Shergill SS, et al: A systematic review of the effects of low-frequency repetitive transcranial magnetic stimulation on cognition. J Neural Transm (Vienna) 123(12):1479–1490, 2016 27503083

Leuchter AF, Cook IA, Feifel D, et al: Efficacy and safety of low-field synchronized transcranial magnetic stimulation (sTMS) for treatment of major depression. Brain Stimul 8(4):787–794, 2015 26143022

Levkovitz Y, Isserles M, Padberg F, et al: Efficacy and safety of deep transcranial magnetic stimulation for major depression: a prospective multicenter randomized controlled trial. World Psychiatry 14(1):64–73, 2015 25655160

Magnezi R, Aminov E, Shmuel D, et al: Comparison between neurostimulation techniques repetitive transcranial magnetic stimulation vs electroconvulsive therapy for the treatment of resistant depression: patient preference and cost-effectiveness. Patient Prefer Adherence 10(10):1481–1487, 2016 27536079

Oberman L, Edwards D, Eldaief M, et al: Safety of theta burst transcranial magnetic stimulation: a systematic review of the literature. J Clin Neurophysiol 28(1):67–74, 2011 21221011

O'Reardon JP, Solvason HB, Janicak PG, et al: Efficacy and safety of transcranial magnetic stimulation in the acute treatment of major depression: a multisite randomized controlled trial. Biol Psychiatry 62(11):1208–1216, 2007 17573044

Pereira LS, Muller VT, da Mota GM, et al: Safety of repetitive transcranial magnetic stimulation in patients with epilepsy: a systematic review. Epilepsy Behav 57 (Pt A):167–176, 2016 26970993

Perera T, George MS, Grammer G, et al: The Clinical TMS Society consensus review and treatment recommendations for TMS therapy for major depression. Brain Stimul 9(3):336–346, 2016 27090022

Rossi S, Hallett M, Rossini PM, et al; Safety of TMS Consensus Group: Safety, ethical considerations, and application guidelines for the use of transcranial magnetic stimulation in clinical practice and research. Clin Neurophysiol 120(12):2008–2039, 2009 19833552

Rossi S, Hallett M, Rossini PM, et al: Screening questionnaire before TMS: an update. Clin Neurophysiol 122(8):1686, 2011 21227747

Schulze L, Wheeler S, McAndrews MP, et al: Cognitive safety of dorsomedial prefrontal repetitive transcranial magnetic stimulation in major depression. Eur Neuropsychopharmacol 26(7):1213–1226, 2016 27157074

Tringali S, Perrot X, Collet L, et al: Repetitive transcranial magnetic stimulation: hearing safety considerations. Brain Stimulat 5(3):354–363, 2012 21824837

Xia G, Gajwani P, Muzina DJ, et al: Treatment-emergent mania in unipolar and bipolar depression: focus on repetitive transcranial magnetic stimulation. Int J Neuropsychopharmacol 11(1):119–130, 2008 17335643

Combining Pharmacotherapy With Transcranial Magnetic Stimulation in the Treatment of Major Depression

Mehmet E. Dokucu, M.D., Ph.D.
Philip G. Janicak, M.D.

The high prevalence of treatment-resistant depression (TRD) has been an important impetus in the development of transcranial magnetic stimulation (TMS). To adequately demonstrate the efficacy of TMS in treating TRD, the pivotal trials included patients treated with TMS monotherapy or sham TMS. The U.S. Food and Drug Administration (FDA) advises that TMS is for treating patients who have experienced one or more failed antidepressant medication trials and who are not presently undergoing any antidepressant therapy. In clinical practice, however, most patients continue taking their antidepressant and other psychotropic medications while receiving an acute course of TMS. Also, after completion of an acute TMS treatment course, the most common maintenance strategy utilizes antidepressant(s) (with or without reintroduction of TMS with impending relapse). In support of this practice, the consensus review of the Clinical TMS Society states that "TMS therapy can be administered with or without the concomitant administration of antidepressant or other psychotropic medications.... [T]here is currently no evidence of an increased risk of adverse events by combining medications with TMS" (Perera et al. 2016, p. 344). According to a survey of Clinical TMS Society members, the majority of practitioners recommend continuing medications during acute TMS therapy and refraining from medication changes during the acute course (Perera et al. 2016).

The choice of medication to combine with TMS to optimize outcome remains problematic. A large number of preclinical and human studies have attempted to elucidate the pathophysiology of depression, as well as antidepressant medication mechanisms. Far fewer studies have attempted to understand the mechanisms of action of device-based treatments such as electroconvulsive therapy, deep brain stimulation, and TMS. A detailed review of these areas of research is beyond the scope of this chapter. It can, however, be confidently stated that due to the heterogeneity of depressive syndromes and lack of consistent biological markers, there are no depression treatments that are based on well-described disease mechanisms. For example, despite the fact that electroconvulsive therapy is very effective and has been available for over 75 years, its use is affected by problems of access, stigma, and tolerability, and its mechanism of action is still not clearly understood, although promising theories are proposed (Kellner et al. 2012). This lack of understanding of the mechanism of action is also true for other forms of therapeutic neuromodulation, and as a result, it is currently not possible to make precise statements about the interaction between TMS and pharmacotherapy when administered concurrently or sequentially during the treatment of depression.

In this chapter, we review the knowledge base and recommended clinical practices for utilizing TMS in combination with pharmacotherapy for acute treatment, sequentially when transitioning from acute

TMS therapy to maintenance medication therapy, and again in combination if TMS reintroduction is needed during the maintenance period.

Augmentation Studies Combining Medication and TMS

ACUTE STUDIES

Many early TMS studies have essentially been augmentation trials because patients were also taking one or more medications. For example, Conca et al. (1996) administered 10 sessions of low-frequency TMS to 12 patients taking antidepressants and compared the results with those of 12 patients who received only medication. Statistically significant changes in scores on the Hamilton Depression Rating Scale (HDRS) favored TMS augmentation after three sessions of TMS ($P<0.003$), and changes were even greater after the tenth session ($P<0.001$). The same research group performed a brief course of 10-day add-on TMS in 12 inpatients and reported that eight subjects (66.7%) responded to the treatment as assessed by HDRS change scores (Conca et al. 2000). They also observed an earlier onset of response in the TMS group (statistical analysis not made available) and proposed that a shorter duration of the index depressive episode may be a positive predictor of treatment response. In a more recent, open-label study, Berlim et al. (2014) used deep TMS as an augmentation to medications. Seventeen outpatients with severe TRD received 4 weeks of daily, high-frequency deep TMS. At week 5, on the basis of HDRS change scores, the remission rate was 41.2% and response rate was 70.6%. For the group receiving TMS, suicidality ($P<0.019$), anxiety ($P<0.0001$), and quality-of-life ($P<0.028$) scores also significantly improved from baseline.

Although TMS has not been approved by the FDA for treating bipolar disorder, many patients are receiving off-label TMS for the depressed phase of the disorder (see Chapter 8, "Transcranial Magnetic Stimulation for the Treatment of Other Mood Disorders"). An add-on safety and feasibility trial ($N=19$) with deep TMS in patients with bipolar depression found a significant decrease from baseline HDRS scores ($P<0.001$) and good tolerability (Harel et al. 2011).

Carpenter et al. (2012) reported the results of a large open-label, naturalistic, acute trial to inform clinicians using TMS in routine practice settings. Forty-two mostly private clinical centers participated. The primary outcome measure was the Clinical Global Impression—Severity of Illness Scale (CGI-S) change score, and the secondary outcomes were change scores on the Inventory of Depressive Symptomatology—Self

Report (IDS-SR) and the 9-item Patient Health Questionnaire (PHQ-9). Nearly all patients continued taking their current psychiatric medications. On the basis of the CGI-S change scores at the end of acute TMS therapy, more than half of the patients met response criteria and approximately one-third achieved remission. Notably, there was no increase in adverse effects.

Su et al. (2005) studied 30 Chinese patients with TRD in a sham-controlled, double-blind, randomized trial in which a 10-session TMS course was added to ongoing medications. Ten participants were assigned to each of three groups, which were assigned to receive either 20-Hz TMS, 5-Hz TMS, or sham TMS. As indicated by HDRS change scores, response rates for patients in the two active TMS arms were superior to those for patients receiving the sham procedure ($P<0.01$; Su et al. 2005).

An ongoing 8-week, multicenter, randomized open-label study titled Augmentation versus Switch: Comparative Effectiveness Research Trial for Antidepressant Incomplete and Non-responders With Treatment Resistant Depression (ASCERTAIN-TRD; https://clinicaltrials.gov, identifier #NCT02977299) will attempt to evaluate TMS versus aripiprazole as augmentation strategies with venlafaxine as the primary treatment. The three open-label arms will consist of 1) aripiprazole augmentation (a 5-mg/day starting dose with a 15-mg/day maximum), 2) TMS augmentation, and 3) switching to venlafaxine extended-release. The primary outcome measure will be the Montgomery-Åsberg Depression Rating Scale (MADRS) change score, and an important secondary outcome will be the Quality of Life Enjoyment and Satisfaction Questionnaire—Short Form (Q-LES-Q-SF) change score.

META-ANALYSES OF TMS ACUTE AUGMENTATION STUDIES

A meta-analysis of sham-controlled clinical trials considered response in patients with TRD using TMS as an augmentation to medication (Liu et al. 2014). Seven randomized trials met the investigators' inclusion criteria, with a total sample size of 279 (171 active TMS patients and 108 sham TMS patients). The response rate was 46.6% for active TMS versus 22.1% for sham TMS (odds ratio=5.12; 95% confidence interval=2.11–12.45; $z=3.60$; $P<0.0003$). The change in baseline HDRS scores also suggested that active TMS was superior to the sham procedure (a small difference of 0.86; $P<0.00001$). The small number of studies and subgroup heterogeneity, however, tempered the authors' conclusions. The results of an earlier meta-analysis (Berlim et al. 2013), which included six studies

(N=392), were consistent with these results. Berlim and colleagues commented that high-frequency TMS may also accelerate time to antidepressant response.

MAINTENANCE AUGMENTATION STUDIES

The pivotal monotherapy TMS trial that led to FDA clearance of the first device for treatment of unipolar major depression included a 6-month durability-of-effect phase. During this period, TMS could be reintroduced as an augmentation to maintenance antidepressant monotherapy. Eighty-four percent (32/38) of patients with predefined worsening of depression for 2 consecutive weeks benefited from reintroduction of TMS (requiring an average of ~14 sessions), with no increase in adverse events (Janicak et al. 2010; O'Reardon et al. 2007).

Phase III of the randomized sham-controlled National Institute of Mental Health–sponsored optimization of TMS (OPT-TMS) study involved medicated and unmedicated patients who achieved remission after Phases I and II of the study. Although participants were followed for 6 months, only the 3-month analysis was performed because of attrition. Approximately half of the patients who achieved remission were taking medication, typically venlafaxine or nortriptyline combined with lithium or lamotrigine. Medicated and unmedicated patient groups did not show any significant difference in clinical outcome at the 3-month follow-up. Fifty-eight percent of the participants were still in remission at 3 months, and 13.5% of the patients had relapsed. Average time to relapse was 7.2 weeks (Mantovani et al. 2012).

The largest maintenance study to date extended to 12 months and included 275 patients with TRD at the end of the acute phase, summarized in "Acute Studies" earlier in this section (Carpenter et al. 2012; Dunner et al. 2014). At the end of the study, 120 patients achieved response or remission and were offered maintenance medication or naturalistic follow-up with the choice of reintroduction of TMS therapy if symptoms worsened. Sixty-two percent of the participants maintained at least response status throughout the 52-week follow-up. Dunner and colleagues concluded that TMS can achieve durability of benefit in a statistically significant ($P<0.0001$) and clinically meaningful way. Of note, 32.5% required a mean number of 16.2 sessions of reintroduction TMS within 1 month of initiating their maintenance phase. Similar to the acute-phase naturalistic study, almost all patients were taking concomitant medications, and the median number of medications was one for remitters and two for the rest of the cohort. No meaningful associations were reported with medication use characteristics and categorical outcomes.

Clinical Considerations When Combining TMS With Medications

ASSESSMENT OF MEDICATION TIMELINE, BENEFITS, AND ADVERSE EFFECTS

During the initial TMS consultation, the clinician should obtain a comprehensive history of antidepressant medications. Although cumbersome to use, the Antidepressant Treatment History Form (ATHF) is one tool that can help gather this information (Sackeim 2001). Although this history is taken primarily to establish the level of treatment resistance, the data can also help inform pharmacotherapy treatment decisions while TMS therapy is in progress. All concomitant psychotropic medications should be carefully categorized as partially helpful or not helpful. Medications that are not at least partially helpful should be sequentially tapered and stopped. Medications that are contributing to adverse effects (e.g., weight gain) and have not been helpful should be tapered first. Ideally, a patient's medication regimen should be stable for at least 2–4 weeks prior to starting TMS; this preparation allows the physician to specifically assess the adverse effects and response to TMS.

Obtaining a list of all current medications, their dosages, and their duration of treatment is critical to understanding and minimizing the risk of seizures. In addition, some medications (e.g., benzodiazepines, high-dose anticonvulsants) may diminish the efficacy of TMS therapy by increasing the activation thresholds of the neuronal circuits (Li et al. 2004). Finally, if patients should report adverse effects that do not commonly occur during TMS, full knowledge of current medications and their timeline may help identify the source more accurately.

RISK FOR SYMPTOM WORSENING WITH MEDICATION CHANGES DURING TMS

Some patients would like to discontinue their current psychiatric medications when they present for a consultation session and will seek the opinion of the TMS clinician. The most common reasons for this desire for discontinuation are medication-related adverse events and a lack of confidence in the effectiveness of one or more medications. Importantly, patients may minimize symptomatic improvements when they initially start the medication. Without a detailed understanding of current medications and the temporal relationship with any changes in symptoms, the TMS clinician cannot formulate an opinion. Furthermore, if the TMS clinician is not the patient's primary mental health care provider, direct communication with that provider is essential in formulating a plan about any medication changes that may enhance the efficacy of TMS, decrease the risk for adverse events, or both. Reviewing records and communicating with the patient's primary treatment team and family can help clarify whether certain medications are partially effective. The fact that patients may not see their primary psychiatric providers during the TMS course increases the importance of the TMS clinician being familiar with the medication regimen and response history.

MEDICATIONS THAT MAY INCREASE TMS-RELATED SEIZURES

Table 4–1 lists the most recent Safety of TMS Consensus Group guidelines for medications that may worsen the seizure risk associated with TMS treatment (Rossi et al. 2009). Although many antidepressants can lower seizure threshold, bupropion carries a more prominent warning regarding its seizure-inducing potential. Hence, we will review it in more detail.

Bupropion, compared with other medications, has lower risks of sexual dysfunction and weight gain and therefore is commonly prescribed as a monotherapy or augmenting agent for patients being treated for depression. This agent, however, carries an increased seizure risk in special populations (i.e., those with eating disorders or those with prior seizure history) and also may alter the motor threshold (Mufti et al. 2010). At times, TMS candidates and their referring clinicians may ask whether it is safe to continue bupropion during TMS therapy. In regard to this issue, one systematic literature review (Dobek et al. 2015) identified 25 TMS-induced seizures between 1980 and 2015, none of which were related to taking bupropion. One patient whose TMS-induced seizure was reported to the FDA was concomitantly taking bupropion, sertraline, and amphetamine. Dobek and colleagues, however, stated that rarely occurring seizures during TMS did not point to a specific antidepressant such as bupropion. Janicak et al. (2008) reported on 34 patients who were taking bupropion and underwent more than 1,000 TMS treatments without a seizure event.

CLINICAL VIGNETTE

The patient is a 27-year-old resident physician who presented for TMS therapy to manage his 4-month treatment-resistant major depressive episode and comorbid migraines. A comprehensive medication history was obtained, and the patient's primary psychiatrist was contacted for verifi-

Table 4–1. Concomitant medications and seizure risk safety classifications, adapted from Safety of TMS Consensus Group guidelines

Strong risk with intake of agent (perform TMS with *particular* caution)	Relative risk with intake of agent (perform TMS with caution)	Relative risk with withdrawal from agent (perform TMS with caution)
Antidepressants	Antidepressants and mood stabilizers	Anticonvulsants and mood stabilizers
Imipramine	Mianserin	Benzodiazepines
Amitriptyline	Fluoxetine	Lamotrigine
Doxepin	Fluvoxamine	Divalproex
Nortriptyline	Paroxetine	Phenytoin
Maprotiline	Sertraline	Sedatives and anxiolytics
Amphetamines	Citalopram	Benzodiazepines
Antipsychotics	Mirtazapine	Barbiturates
Chlorpromazine	Reboxetine	Meprobamate
Clozapine	Bupropion	Chloral hydrate
Drugs of abuse	Lithium	Drugs of abuse
Alcohol	Antipsychotics	Alcohol
Amphetamines	Fluphenazine	Benzodiazepines
Ketamine	Pimozide	Barbiturates

Table 4–1. Concomitant medications and seizure risk safety classifications, adapted from Safety of TMS Consensus Group guidelines *(continued)*

Strong risk with intake of agent (perform TMS with particular caution)	Relative risk with intake of agent (perform TMS with caution)	Relative risk with withdrawal from agent (perform TMS with caution)
Phencyclidine	Haloperidol	
Cocaine	Olanzapine	
γ-Hydroxybutyrate	Quetiapine	
3,4-Methylenedioxymethamphetamine (MDMA; Ecstasy)	Aripiprazole	
	Ziprasidone	
Other	Risperidone	
Foscarnet	Other	
Theophylline	Chloroquine	
Ganciclovir	Mefloquine	
	Imipenem	
	Penicillin	
	Ampicillin	

Table 4–1. Concomitant medications and seizure risk safety classifications, adapted from Safety of TMS Consensus Group guidelines (continued)

Strong risk with intake of agent (perform TMS with *particular caution*)	Relative risk with intake of agent (perform TMS with caution)	Relative risk with withdrawal from agent (perform TMS with caution)
	Cephalosporins	
	Metronidazole	
	Isoniazid	
	Levofloxacin	
	Cyclosporine	
	Chlorambucil	
	Vincristine	
	Methotrexate	
	Cytosine arabinoside	
	Bis-chloroethylnitrosourea	
	Anticholinergics	
	Antihistamines	
	Sympathomimetics	

Note. TMS=transcranial magnetic stimulation.
Source. Adapted from Rossi et al. 2009.

cation. He was taking bupropion extended-release 450 mg/day, which was initiated after his poor tolerance of two selective serotonin reuptake inhibitors and one serotonin-norepinephrine reuptake inhibitor because of sexual dysfunction and increased appetite and associated weight gain. The bupropion daily dose was titrated from 150 mg to 450 mg because of gradual but small improvement of his depressive symptoms. Even at 450 mg, however, he continued to experience functional impairment as well as dose-related worsening of his migraines. He began undergoing left dorsolateral prefrontal cortex high-frequency (10 Hz) TMS therapy, and over the course of 2 weeks, his bupropion was tapered to 150 mg, with complete resolution of his migraines. He continued TMS for another 4 weeks, ultimately achieving complete remission of depressive symptoms, with a final IDS-SR score of 6 (down from a baseline score of 53). Furthermore, the patient experienced no significant adverse effects with the combination of bupropion and TMS.

MEDICATIONS THAT MAY COMPROMISE TMS EFFICACY

Although some TMS practitioners express concern that concomitant use of benzodiazepines or other anticonvulsants may compromise efficacy and/or alter TMS dose requirements, the existing literature does not support this contention (Ziemann 2013). Nevertheless, if physicians believe that these medications should be lowered or tapered prior to or during the initial weeks of TMS therapy, care must be taken not to abruptly stop them, which can increase seizure risk, particularly in patients with epilepsy.

MEDICATIONS TO MINIMIZE RISKS ASSOCIATED WITH TMS

Severe insomnia, at times resulting in sleep deprivation, can significantly increase seizure risk during TMS therapy. This risk can be attenuated by treatment of insomnia with agents such as ramelteon, trazodone, zolpidem, zaleplon, eszopiclone, or, less desirably, short-half-life benzodiazepines. If available, cognitive-behavioral therapy for insomnia may be the preferred option.

On occasion, some patients who have significant anxiety and/or restlessness may find it difficult to sit still for the duration of a TMS therapy session. Such patients can be premedicated with low doses of quetiapine, diphenhydramine, or hydroxyzine if their restlessness is not responsive to changes in their scheduled medications.

It is acceptable but not commonly needed for patients to take over-the-counter nonsteroidal anti-inflammatory drugs prior to their sessions to decrease scalp discomfort or headaches. Very rarely, more severe discomfort may require and typically responds to local anesthetics (e.g., topical skin preparations).

Conclusion

Although TMS is an effective and safe treatment for major depression, it is still in its earlier stages of development and refinement. In this light, the available preclinical and clinical data to guide decisions about combining or sequencing TMS with pharmacotherapy should be considered preliminary. For now, most patients in clinical practice usually receive concurrent medications with no apparent compromise in efficacy or increase in adverse events. Ongoing research and clinical experience will undoubtedly facilitate the development of future combination protocols that can safely enhance the effectiveness of treatment. For example, although investigational at this time, TMS augmentation strategies using agents such as ketamine and related compounds may represent viable strategies to manage more resistant depressions and/or hasten the onset of efficacy.

KEY CLINICAL POINTS

- TMS monotherapy is effective for major depression.

- Augmentation of TMS with antidepressants and/or other psychotropic medications is frequently used in clinical practice and may enhance overall benefit.

- The role for TMS augmentation strategies is supported by large acute studies and maintenance studies conducted under naturalistic conditions.

- There is preliminary evidence to support the off-label use of TMS combined with various mood stabilizers for bipolar depression.

- Because most patients in clinical practice receive psychotropic medications plus TMS, heightened awareness for potential changes in efficacy and risks is required.

- The prescription of medications with TMS requires the psychopharmacologist and TMS physician to communicate clearly and clarify the roles and responsibilities of each professional.

References

Berlim MT, Van den Eynde F, Daskalakis ZJ: High-frequency repetitive transcranial magnetic stimulation accelerates and enhances the clinical response to antidepressants in major depression: a meta-analysis of randomized, double-blind, and sham-controlled trials. J Clin Psychiatry 74(2):e122–e129, 2013 23473357

Berlim MT, Van den Eynde F, Tovar-Perdomo S, et al: Augmenting antidepressants with deep transcranial magnetic stimulation (DTMS) in treatment-resistant major depression. World J Biol Psychiatry 15(7):570–578, 2014 25050453

Carpenter LL, Janicak PG, Aaronson ST, et al: Transcranial magnetic stimulation (TMS) for major depression: a multisite, naturalistic, observational study of acute treatment outcomes in clinical practice. Depress Anxiety 29(7):587–596, 2012 22689344

Conca A, Coppi S, König P, et al: Transcranial magnetic stimulation: a novel antidepressive strategy. Neuropsychobiology 34(4):204–207, 1996 9121622

Conca A, Swoboda E, König P, et al: Clinical impacts of single transcranial magnetic stimulation (sTMS) as an add-on therapy in severely depressed patients under SSRI treatment. Hum Psychopharmacol 15(6):429–438, 2000 12404305

Dobek CE, Blumberger DM, Downar J, et al: Risk of seizures in transcranial magnetic stimulation: a clinical review to inform consent process focused on bupropion. Neuropsychiatr Dis Treat 11:2975–2987, 2015 26664122

Dunner DL, Aaronson ST, Sackeim HA, et al: A multisite, naturalistic, observational study of transcranial magnetic stimulation for patients with pharmacoresistant major depressive disorder: durability of benefit over a 1-year follow-up period. J Clin Psychiatry 75(12):1394–1401, 2014 25271871

Harel EV, Zangen A, Roth Y, et al: H-coil repetitive transcranial magnetic stimulation for the treatment of bipolar depression: an add-on, safety and feasibility study. World J Biol Psychiatry 12(2):119–126, 2011 20854181

Janicak PG, O'Reardon JP, Sampson SM, et al: Transcranial magnetic stimulation in the treatment of major depressive disorder: a comprehensive summary of safety experience from acute exposure, extended exposure, and during reintroduction treatment. J Clin Psychiatry 69(2):222–232, 2008 18232722

Janicak PG, Nahas Z, Lisanby SH, et al: Durability of clinical benefit with transcranial magnetic stimulation (TMS) in the treatment of pharmacoresistant major depression: assessment of relapse during a 6-month, multisite, open-label study. Brain Stimulat 3(4):187–199, 2010 20965447

Kellner CH, Greenberg RM, Murrough JW, et al: ECT in treatment-resistant depression. Am J Psychiatry 169(12):1238–1244, 2012 23212054

Li X, Tenebäck CC, Nahas Z, et al: Interleaved transcranial magnetic stimulation/functional MRI confirms that lamotrigine inhibits cortical excitability in healthy young men. Neuropsychopharmacology 29(7):1395–1407, 2004 15100699

Liu B, Zhang Y, Zhang L, Li L: Repetitive transcranial magnetic stimulation as an augmentative strategy for treatment-resistant depression, a meta-analysis of randomized, double-blind and sham-controlled study. BMC Psychiatry 14:342, 2014 25433539

Mantovani A, Pavlicova M, Avery D, et al: Long-term efficacy of repeated daily prefrontal transcranial magnetic stimulation (TMS) in treatment-resistant depression. Depress Anxiety 29(10):883–890, 2012 22689290

Mufti MA, Holtzheimer PE, Epstein CM, et al: Bupropion decreases resting motor threshold: a case report. Brain Stimul 3(3):177–180, 2010 20633447

O'Reardon JP, Solvason HB, Janicak PG, et al: Efficacy and safety of transcranial magnetic stimulation in the acute treatment of major depression: a multisite randomized controlled trial. Biol Psychiatry 62(11):1208–1216, 2007 17573044

Perera T, George MS, Grammer G, et al: The Clinical TMS Society Consensus Review and Treatment Recommendations for TMS Therapy for Major Depressive Disorder. Brain Stimul 9(3):336–346, 2016 27090022

Rossi S, Hallett M, Rossini PM, et al: Safety of TMS Consensus Group: Safety, ethical considerations, and application guidelines for the use of transcranial magnetic stimulation in clinical practice and research. Clin Neurophysiol 120(12):2008–2039, 2009 19833552

Sackeim HA: The definition and meaning of treatment-resistant depression. J Clin Psychiatry 62 (suppl 16):10–17, 2001 11480879

Su TP, Huang CC, Wei IH: Add-on rTMS for medication-resistant depression: a randomized, double-blind, sham-controlled trial in Chinese patients. J Clin Psychiatry 66(7):930–937, 2005 16013911

Ziemann U: Pharmaco-transcranial magnetic stimulation studies of motor excitability. Handb Clin Neurol 116:387–397, 2013 24112911

5

Transcranial Magnetic Stimulation and Psychotherapy

Sasha Bergeron, M.S.N., PMHNP-BC
Richard A. Bermudes, M.D.

In the overall management of any illness, a clinician should consider an approach that yields high efficacy with comparatively few side effects. Complex psychiatric disorders often require a multimodal treatment model to improve outcomes, especially for patients with treatment-resistant disorders. In this chapter, we review nonpharmacological interventions used in conjunction with transcranial magnetic stimulation (TMS) for the treatment of psychiatric and neurological disorders. A number of studies, ranging from case reports to randomized controlled trials, support the use of such an integrated approach. The combination of TMS with therapeutic interventions is rooted in both practical and biological rationale. We review evidence-based psychotherapies for treatment-resistant depression (TRD) and explore the feasibility of implementing them over the course of TMS therapy. Rather than totally replacing ongoing psychological treatments, TMS should be used in conjunction with other well-established modalities to enhance outcomes for difficult-to-treat populations.

Rationale for Combining TMS and Psychotherapy

One of every four patients with a psychiatric disorder does not adequately respond to or tolerate standard treatment (Bajbouj and Padberg 2014). The burden of insufficiently treated mental illness manifests in decreased quality of life, increased socioeconomic burden, and higher risk of morbidity and mortality. As Bajbouj and Padberg (2014) point out, a multimodal approach should be chosen for patients with treatment-refractory disorders. Although psychotherapy and psychopharmacological combinations are often used together for moderately to severely ill patients, studies find that this approach is not effective for about 30% of major depressive episodes (Rush et al. 2006; Serafini et al. 2015). Adjunctive brain stimulation interventions may facilitate psychotherapeutic processes and are already being used to treat various psychiatric disorders. Patients are increasingly interested in nonmedication treatments because medications are not always effective and have significant side effects. Additionally, psychotherapeutic treatments may take time to yield effect and can be burdensome on individuals due to the time commitment involved and expensive out-of-pocket costs. It is important to keep in mind, however, that TMS does not replace psychotherapeutic or psychopharmacological interventions; rather, it represents another treatment option as part of a multimodal approach for these complex disorders.

Although psychotherapy is a well-established approach in the treatment of depression, researchers are now investigating whether brain stimulation combined with therapeutic interventions can enhance patient outcomes. Not only does TMS improve depressed mood, but it is also a promising modality to enhance cognition (Guse et al. 2010; Serafini et al. 2015). Evidence suggests that plasticity in the brain in response to stimulation depends on the state of the brain or the activation of the circuit during stimulation, inferring that brain plasticity may be impacted by how activated neural circuits are during TMS sessions (Vedeniapin et al. 2010). There is also evidence that psychotherapy induces neuro-plastic changes in brain function and structure (Figure 5–1). The fact that both modalities have this capacity raises the distinct possibility that engaging the brain via psychotherapy during a TMS session (in which the brain is being stimulated) may magnify the benefits of both treatments. In other words, while undergoing TMS a more engaged brain (i.e., during psychotherapy) may be more receptive to the benefits of TMS than a less engaged brain (i.e., while watching TV). Thus, combining the two interventions may, in fact, have a synergistic effect by modulating mood circuits in complementary ways. Although TMS may prime and/or augment psychotherapy if treatments are administered in succession ("offline" treatment), it is also practical to coadminister psychotherapy during TMS sessions ("online" treatment) because patients are coming to the clinic 5 days/week and on average are in a treatment session for 35–45 minutes. Figure 5–2 provides a visual overview of various ways to administer TMS with psychotherapy.

Can a patient's specific brain state be changed or supported during TMS sessions such that there are improved outcomes? Isserles et al. (2011) hypothesized that the antidepressant outcome of TMS treatment is affected by a cognitive-emotional procedure performed during stimulation. Patients received 4 weeks of daily TMS and 4 weeks of maintenance TMS. Two subgroups of patients received either positive or negative cognitive-emotional reactivation along with the stimulation sessions. These states, either positive or negative, were induced by patients reading short directive paragraphs describing personalized positive or negative emotional states prior to and during the treatments.

Across all of the groups, 21 of 46 patients (46%) who received at least 10 stimulation sessions achieved response (improvement of ≥50% on the Hamilton Depression Rating Scale [HDRS]), and 13 (28%) achieved remission (HDRS ≤10) by the end of the daily treatment phase. Improvements were smaller in the negatively reactivated group, and Beck Depression Inventory (BDI) scores were not significantly improved in this group, signifying that negative cognitive-emotional reactivation may disrupt the therapeutic effects of deep TMS. These results suggest that topics of discussion and focus during TMS treatment sessions may affect response to treatment, although more studies with larger sample sizes are needed. Investigators at Duke University plan to further test this hypothesis by engaging a specific brain network, using cognitive restructuring (a cognitive-behavioral therapy [CBT] technique), and enhancing learning by using TMS (Neacsiu 2015). The results are likely to add to the growing body of evidence that what happens while patients are in the treatment chair impacts treatment outcomes.

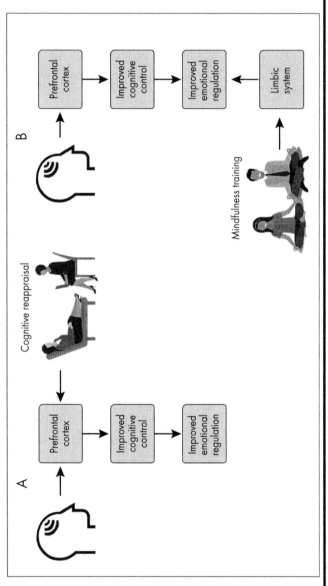

Figure 5–1. Psychotherapy and transcranial magnetic stimulation induction of neuroplastic changes that normalize neural networks instrumental in mood regulation.

(A) Theoretically, psychotherapy and transcranial magnetic stimulation (TMS) may be combined to target prefrontal cortex function, resulting in improved cognitive control and improved emotional regulation ("top down"). (B) Certain psychotherapeutic practices may target limbic network functioning and may be combined with TMS, resulting in improved emotional functioning ("bottom up" and "top down").

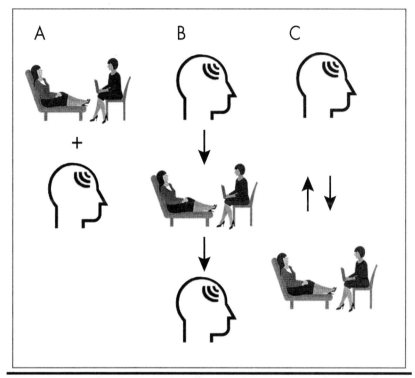

Figure 5–2. "Online" and "offline" administration of psychotherapy plus transcranial magnetic stimulation.

Transcranial magnetic stimulation and psychotherapy can be administered (A) during the same session ("online"); (B) sequentially, so as to prime one intervention ("offline"); or (C) randomly, but during the same treatment course ("offline").

CLINICAL VIGNETTE

The patient is a 57-year-old man receiving bilateral TMS for his severe, recurrent TRD and comorbid generalized anxiety disorder. He previously underwent two courses of CBT and multiple antidepressant medication trials, each of which was ineffective. Over the course of his TMS treatment (42 sessions total), he received concurrent psychotherapy during his TMS sessions one to two times weekly ("online" treatment) as well as one "offline" session weekly that occurred either immediately before or after a TMS session. His treatment provider administered psychotherapy and managed the psychotropic medications. Various therapeutic modalities that were incorporated into sessions included behavioral activation and cognitive restructuring (a CBT approach); relaxation training using a progressive muscle relaxation exercise; problem-focused therapy to correct sleep and appetite disturbances; mindfulness meditation techniques, such as awareness of breath and purposeful attention to the present moment; and supportive therapy, including empathetic listening, reassurance, and encouragement.

Practical implementation involved the selection of specific, effective therapeutic interventions. The components necessary to foster a good therapeutic rapport included eye contact, positioning, volume of speech, and privacy. These were maintained utilizing a variety of techniques: The provider sat directly in front of the patient, at a height that was comfortable to maintain eye contact, because the patient was in a fixed position during treatment. Both the provider and the patient were sensitive to the auditory interruptions of the TMS pulse trains, and during the right-sided low-frequency treatment (1 pulse per second), each spoke at a slightly higher than normal amplitude over the metronomic pulse delivery. For the left-sided high-frequency treatment (10 pulses per second for 4 seconds), speech was paused, even if mid-sentence, and resumed during the intertrain interval (10 seconds). Privacy was maintained with white noise machines throughout the office. The patient agreed to participate in therapy knowing a technician would be present; the technician maintained discretion during sessions and had a good rapport with the patient. Ultimately, the patient achieved a 63% reduction in depressive symptoms as measured by the 9-item Patient Health Questionnaire (PHQ-9) and a 66% reduction in anxiety symptoms as measured by the Generalized Anxiety Disorder 7-item scale (GAD-7). In his final session, the patient reflected that the combination of psychotherapy and TMS was particularly helpful in identifying triggers and improving coping skills. In summary, practical barriers to implementing concurrent TMS and psychotherapy were easily identified and adjusted to provide a successful course of "online" therapy with TMS.

Though more research is needed on the topic, evidence is building that this simultaneous treatment approach may have enhanced outcomes for a patient with severe TRD.

Review of Literature

Although the benefits of combining TMS and psychotherapy are promising, the use of TMS in conjunction with psychotherapy has not been well studied. It is not clear whether patients in outpatient, open-label effectiveness trials (Carpenter et al. 2012) received psychotherapy while in treatment. In our own TMS centers, the decision to combine psychotherapy with TMS is an individualized treatment decision. We find that some patients prefer to temporarily stop psychotherapy because of the time commitment with TMS, whereas others who have started to benefit from TMS resume therapy and report improved effectiveness. Nonetheless, a literature review of TMS and psychotherapy provides insight into this promising multimodal approach. Although many questions remain unanswered, a growing body of evidence supports coalescing

Table 5–1. Overview of psychotherapeutic modalities used with transcranial magnetic stimulation (TMS) for various disorders

Condition	Therapy	Delivery	Reference
Depression	Cognitive-behavioral therapy	Online	Vedeniapin et al. 2010
Posttraumatic stress disorder	Exposure therapy	Online	Osuch et al. 2009
Obsessive-compulsive disorder	Exposure and response prevention therapy	Offline	Grassi et al. 2015
Poststroke	Speech and language therapy	Offline	Yoon et al. 2015
	Virtual reality training	Online	Zheng et al. 2015
	Occupational therapy	Offline	Kakuda et al. 2010
Alzheimer's disease	Cognitive training	Offline	Rabey et al. 2013

Note. Online=therapy delivered simultaneously with TMS treatment; offline=therapy delivered outside of TMS treatment session but over the course of TMS treatment.

therapeutic modalities and TMS for both psychiatric and neurological disorders. Table 5–1 provides an overview of the various therapeutic modalities studied in combination with TMS.

TMS AND PSYCHOTHERAPY FOR MAJOR DEPRESSIVE DISORDER

Although research combining TMS with psychotherapy for the treatment of major depression is limited, there is a case report describing the use of CBT with TMS in a patient with TRD. Vedeniapin et al. (2010) treated a female patient who had severe TRD with simultaneous CBT and left prefrontal TMS ("online" treatment). Prior to the study, the patient had responded to a course of TMS, but a mild relapse 1 year later necessitated a subsequent series of 14 TMS sessions. Symptoms gradually worsened again, even with medication management and weekly psychotherapy. At the time of this study, the patient's depressive symptoms were severe. She was first educated on the basics of CBT and then received 14 excitatory (10 Hz) TMS-CBT sessions, interspersed with 25 TMS-only sessions over an 8-week course of treatment. She experienced a gradual reduction in symptoms, ultimately achieving remission, with fewer sessions overall during this course of treatment (39 total sessions) than in her initial course of TMS (59 total sessions). She maintained remission for at least 3 months. This case report suggests that CBT can be combined with TMS to improve symptoms and maintain remission from depression, although more research with controlled studies is needed (Vedeniapin et al. 2010).

Functional neuroimaging research suggests that mindfulness exercises activate a number of brain structures implicated in regulating emotions and reappraisal, including the dorsolateral prefrontal cortex (DLPFC) (Chiesa et al. 2013; Ochsner et al. 2002). A related question is whether TMS can be used to prime for psychotherapeutic interventions. In a retrospective chart review, Leong et al. (2013) examined the change in four components of mindfulness in individuals with major depression who had received a course of TMS. The investigators reported that patients' scores significantly improved on the Nonreactivity to Inner Experience subscale of Baer's Five Facet Mindfulness Questionnaire (BFFMQ) ($P<0.05$) and on the Decentering subscale of the Experience Questionnaire (EQ) ($P<0.05$). Of note, scores on these components of mindfulness showed improvement after TMS and were independent of changes in depression scores. The subjects showed improvement in emotional regulation normally seen in individuals who practice mindfulness. Although in this study mindfulness exercises were not prescribed during the TMS treatment course, one wonders if the combination of TMS and mindfulness may enhance or speed up achieving better emotional regulation. Referring practitioners may consider prescribing mindfulness exercises to be used alongside a course of TMS therapy.

TMS AND PSYCHOTHERAPY FOR OTHER PSYCHIATRIC DISORDERS

Evidence is emerging regarding the benefits of using psychotherapy and TMS to treat disorders other than major depressive disorder. For example, Marin and Milad (2015) hypothesized that augmentation with TMS could facilitate the consolidation process of learning during exposure-based therapies and improve responses for patients with treatment-resistant posttraumatic stress disorder (PTSD). In a crossover study, Osuch et al. (2009) randomly assigned nine adults with treatment-refractory PTSD to imaginal exposure therapy combined with 1-Hz TMS over the right DLPFC or a sham procedure. Prior to treatment, patients developed an individual exposure hierarchy consisting of 10 cues for use during sessions. The hierarchy began with an item 0, chosen by the subject to be calming, with subsequent experiences eliciting incrementally increasing levels of distress. During the sessions, patients could control how much of the traumatic experience they were exposed to, could talk about any of the traumatic cues, or could remain silent. All patients completed the 4-week protocol of imaginal exposure therapy during TMS ("online" therapy). Although this was a small study, active TMS treatment showed a large, but not significant, effect on hyperarousal symptoms compared with sham TMS ($P=0.08$). Furthermore, 24-hour urinary norepinephrine and serum thyroxine levels increased, and prolactin levels decreased. The authors concluded that TMS therapy with imaginal exposure therapy was well tolerated and feasible and had symptomatic as well as physiological effects in patients with severe, treatment-refractory PTSD (Osuch et al. 2009). These results, although preliminary, support conducting larger studies in the future to clarify the effects of combining exposure therapy with TMS for PTSD.

In an individual case report, TMS enhanced the results of exposure and response prevention therapy for a patient with treatment-resistant obsessive-compulsive disorder (OCD) (Grassi et al. 2015). The subject in this report was a 32-year-old woman with severe OCD (since age 10) and concurrent mild depression. She experienced a low level of daily functioning and had failed to respond to multiple serotonergic drugs, augmentation with second-generation atypical antipsychotics, and two different CBT trials at specialized OCD centers. As described in this case report, she underwent 16 sessions of CBT, with the latter 10 centered on exposure and response prevention exercises. Prior to each exposure session, she was given a high-frequency TMS session over the left DLPFC. A score reduction of 32.14% from her baseline score on the Yale-Brown Obsessive Compulsive Scale (Y-BOCS) was observed after the final treatment session and was maintained at 6-, 12-, and 24-month follow-ups. The patient also reported significantly improved quality of life and daily functioning. Grassi et al. (2015) concluded that TMS might enhance extinction learning because of its durable effects on neuroplasticity, although further systematic studies are required to establish reliability.

TMS AND REHABILITATIVE THERAPIES FOR NEUROCOGNITIVE DISORDERS

In addition to being combined with psychotherapy, TMS can be combined with other nonpharmacological interventions to treat various neurocognitive disorders. Neurocognitive illnesses and injuries are disabling and negatively impact physical functioning, mental capacity, relationships, and employment. Furthermore, standard treatments such as rehabilitative therapy and pharmacological treatment rendered in community settings do not fully restore affected patients. Research has recently examined the combination of TMS with rehabilitative therapies to treat neurocognitive disorders. Table 5–2 provides an overview of the literature on integrating TMS with rehabilitative therapies in the treatment of select neurocognitive disorders.

Combining Therapy, Behavioral Skills, and Exercises With TMS

There are several depression-specific therapies and behavioral skills that can be combined with TMS both during and outside of treatment sessions (Strunk 2017). As highlighted earlier, when psychotherapies or exercises are prescribed outside of the TMS therapy session, they are referred to as "offline" interventions, but when administered during the TMS therapy session, they are referred to as "online" interventions. Behavioral activation, cognitive therapy, and interpersonal psychotherapy have strong research support as monotherapies for patients with depression. These treatments are used in clinical practice and should be thought of as optimal modalities to combine with TMS for patients with TRD.

Before therapy is initiated, it is important to understand the patient's history of therapy; this helps to determine the individual's level of treatment resistance and provides an inventory of prior therapies. Histories should document the approximate start and stop dates of treatment, frequency of sessions, type of psychotherapy or skills taught, treatment focus, and therapist's name and degree. If validated instruments were used to measure change in depressive symptoms, then pretreatment and posttreatment scores should be documented. Patients can usually report a subjective sense of whether a treatment was helpful, partially helpful, or unhelpful. Some patients are hesitant to restart therapy or continue therapy in conjunction with TMS because they may have a perception that therapy "did not work" or may reference time constraints as a barrier to pursing both treatments. Building motivation, establishing goals, and exploring negative perceptions about therapy are instrumental for patients to have success when combining TMS with therapy.

Table 5–2. A selective literature review concentrating on transcranial magnetic stimulation (TMS) and rehabilitative therapies in the treatment of neurocognitive disorders

Rehabilitative therapy	Treatment-focused problem	Study design	Methods	Summary of findings
Speech and language therapy (SLT) (Yoon et al. 2015)	Poststroke nonfluent aphasia	Case study	Experimental group ($n=10$): 1-Hz TMS 5 days a week with 2 days followed by SLT for 4 weeks. Control group ($n=10$): SLT 2 times a week for 4 weeks.	TMS+SLT group showed significant improvement over SLT-only group in repetition and naming. TMS prior to SLT could precondition brain to be more responsive to intensive training programs for aphasia and help facilitate neural activity, although more research is required.

Table 5–2. A selective literature review concentrating on transcranial magnetic stimulation (TMS) and rehabilitative therapies in the treatment of neurocognitive disorders (*continued*)

Rehabilitative therapy	Treatment-focused problem	Study design	Methods	Summary of findings
Cognitive training (COG) (Rabey et al. 2013)	Alzheimer's disease (AD)	Double-blind RCT	Treatment group (*n*=7): 1-Hz daily TMS-COG. Control group (*n*=8): sham TMS-COG. Both groups received 5 sessions/week for 6 weeks, followed by biweekly sessions for 3 months.	Primary outcome was significantly improved cognitive scores for the treatment group. Secondary outcomes included significant improvement in score on the Clinical Global Impression of Change (CGIC) and nonsignificant improvement in score on the Neuropsychiatric Inventory (NPI) for the treatment group. TMS-COG was found to be safe and efficacious for improving cognitive function in AD.

Table 5–2. A selective literature review concentrating on transcranial magnetic stimulation (TMS) and rehabilitative therapies in the treatment of neurocognitive disorders *(continued)*

Rehabilitative therapy	Treatment-focused problem	Study design	Methods	Summary of findings
Virtual reality (VR) training (Zheng et al. 2015)	Upper limb functioning for poststroke hemiplegia	Double-blind RCT	Experimental group (*n*=55): low-frequency TMS+VR training. Control group (*n*=53): sham TMS+VR training. Both groups received therapy 6 days/week for 4 weeks.	Upper limb motor function was significantly increased in the experimental group compared with the control group. Results suggest that low-frequency TMS+VR training is a promising rehabilitative treatment for effectively improving upper limb function in patients with hemiplegia following subacute stroke.

Table 5–2. A selective literature review concentrating on transcranial magnetic stimulation (TMS) and rehabilitative therapies in the treatment of neurocognitive disorders *(continued)*

Rehabilitative therapy	Treatment-focused problem	Study design	Methods	Summary of findings
Occupational therapy (OT) (Kakuda et al. 2010)	Upper limb hemiparesis poststroke	Case study	Inpatient combination treatment provided for 5 poststroke patients with upper limb hemiparesis. Over 6 consecutive days, each patient received 10 sessions of 1-Hz TMS and intensive OT.	All patients completed treatment protocol, and none showed adverse effects. At the end of treatment, scores assessing motor function in the affected upper limb had improved in all patients. No deterioration of improved upper limb function was observed at 4 weeks posttreatment. Combination treatment seems safe and feasible, but larger studies are required for validation.

Note. RCT=randomized controlled trial.

"OFFLINE" PSYCHOTHERAPEUTIC INTERVENTIONS AND TMS

CBT is well studied for patients with TRD (Wiles et al. 2013). This approach utilizes a systematic method to analyze and evaluate negative thought patterns. Patients receiving TMS can do cognitive therapy while in treatment (i.e., "online") and over the course of treatment (i.e., "offline"). CBT can also be introduced to patients as they improve over a course of TMS or after they achieve acute response or remission because CBT can support remission maintenance (Biesheuvel-Leliefeld et al. 2015). Basic cognitive and behavioral skills can be taught to patients during a course of TMS therapy with Internet-based programs such as the MoodGYM training program (https://moodgym.com.au). Table 5–3 provides a list of popular computer-based and facilitated psychotherapeutic interventions. For most common anxiety and mood disorders, computer-based CBT programs can be as effective as face-to-face therapy, provided periodic check-ins with a therapist are maintained (Cuijpers et al. 2010). There are also several applications available for mobile phone users based on CBT, and preliminary studies indicate that these applications are comparable to computer-based CBT programs (Watts et al. 2013). In addition, mobile system applications may improve adherence and access, because users can learn or practice skills when it is most convenient for them.

Behavioral activation (BA) is an empirically supported therapy for patients with moderate to severe depression (Strunk 2017). Depressed patients experience decreasing positive emotions in their environments, and in an effort to cope with these negative emotions, they often withdraw and isolate themselves, leading to increased maladaptive behaviors. Through BA, patients identify these behaviors and develop activities and actions that lead to more positive emotions, thus increasing positive reinforcement. BA has research support for its use in both the acute and maintenance phases of depression (Dimidjian et al. 2006; Dobson et al. 2008). BA or behavioral techniques, which target avoidance and withdrawal behaviors, are practical for patients who are "cognitively shut down" by their depression, and they are validated as stand-alone treatments for major depressive disorder. For patients with TRD who are undergoing a course of TMS, BA techniques may be utilized in a variety of ways, including simple coaching by the TMS treatment team and "offline" delivery with a separate therapist.

Mindfulness-based CBT has research support for use with patients with TRD (Eisendrath et al. 2008). It was one of the first therapy systems to demonstrate that patients receiving the treatment, specifically during

Table 5–3. Computer-facilitated psychotherapeutic interventions

Product name	Description	Link
MoodGYM	Free Web-based CBT for depression	https://moodgym.com.au
Headspace	Subscription smartphone/ tablet app; guided meditation for stress and anxiety	www.headspace.com
myCompass	CBT self-help program for managing depression, stress, and anxiety; free and available on any type of device	www.mycompass.org.au
Sleepio	CBT self-help insomnia program; subscription-based program with Internet and mobile applications	www.sleepio.com
E-couch	Free Web-based self-help program for depression and anxiety; draws from CBT and IPT	https://ecouch.anu.edu.au
MoodKit	CBT-based mobile platform for tracking mood and mood-boosting activities and skills	www.thriveport.com

Note.   CBT=cognitive-behavioral therapy; IPT=interpersonal psychotherapy.

the remission phase of depression, had reduced relapse rates compared with patients receiving usual care (Teasdale et al. 2000). Mindfulness-based CBT combines cognitive techniques and mindfulness practices to help patients better recognize catastrophic cognitions regarding their moods, which predispose them to depressive relapse. Patients practice specific exercises and learn to direct their attention to what is happening in the present moment, while taking a nonjudgmental approach to their experiences. Mindfulness-based CBT is becoming more readily available, and there have been several patient self-help books published (e.g., Williams et al. 2007).

Interpersonal therapy (IPT), another modality of psychotherapy, was initially studied for the treatment of major depression. The basis for this therapy lies in the theory that changes in interpersonal relationships often trigger depression. Depressive symptoms can also change or negatively impact interpersonal relationships. Over the course of 12–16 sessions, IPT therapists focus on improving problematic interpersonal relationships that directly relate to the patient's current depressive episode. Patients receiving IPT during the acute phase of depression or after achieving remission have improved durability of remission (Cuijpers et al. 2016). Thus, IPT can be started in conjunction with TMS or after patients have achieved response or remission and are tapering TMS therapy.

There is research supporting the use of IPT for patients with other conditions, such as eating disorders (Cuijpers et al. 2016). Therefore, several clinical considerations may influence the decision to use this therapy, including the impact of depressive symptoms on interpersonal functioning, depression precipitated by a significant interpersonal change, a diagnosis of unipolar or bipolar depression, and comorbidity with an eating disorder. There is also an Internet-based IPT program, E-couch (https://ecouch.anu.edu.au; see Table 5–3), which can be easily incorporated into TMS sessions and reinforced by the TMS treatment team.

Engaging in healthy behaviors and activities between TMS treatment sessions can benefit patients. Table 5–4 lists multiple activities, such as exercise, yoga, and journaling, that can assist the patient in countering the symptomatic isolation and withdrawal of severe depression. Patients can be encouraged by their TMS provider and TMS technician to engage in such activities over the course of TMS therapy. Anecdotally, patients who engage in healthy behaviors early in their treatment course have greater and more durable reductions in depressive symptoms; however, no systematic research has been done on the combination of these activities with TMS.

"ONLINE" PSYCHOTHERAPEUTIC INTERVENTIONS AND TMS

A number of psychotherapeutic interventions can be used by the treatment team during TMS treatment sessions. These include the use of self-help manuals, Internet therapies, and brief coping skills, which may be taught or coached by TMS technicians while the patient is in the TMS chair. These treatments are considered low-tech in the sense that they can be delivered during the treatment session by a TMS technician or with the use of readily accessible technology, such as a TV or tablet. High-tech treatments are less common during the TMS session because they require a licensed therapist trained in depression-specific therapies. Because patients come to treatment 5 days/week for 4–6 weeks, and treatments typically last 35–40 minutes, it is important to plan and

---

Table 5–4. "Offline" therapeutic activities to augment antidepressant effects of transcranial magnetic stimulation

---

Walking at least 30 minutes/day

Yoga

Meditation practice

Hiking

Tennis and other sports

Hobbies such as knitting

Good sleep hygiene

Healthy eating (e.g., reducing or eliminating sugar or gluten)

Joining jogging or running groups

Reestablishing friendships

Journaling

Moderating caffeine and alcohol intake

Increasing natural light exposure

Volunteering/community service

Religious or spiritual activities

---

discuss how to best utilize patients' time in the treatment chair. Each TMS treatment provides an opportunity to use a multimodal treatment approach within the same session ("online"), pairing brain stimulation with daily, assisted therapeutic work.

Internet therapies are widely available and are tools that can be easily incorporated into the TMS treatment room via a smart TV or handheld tablet. TMS technicians can "coach" or cue patients in certain exercises or skills, as prescribed by the treating provider. While in the TMS chair, patients could have the option to complete programs directed at specific diagnoses, such as depression or anxiety, or to select programs targeting specific symptoms, such as sleep or cognitive function. Programs that target anxiety, for example, can be used to address comorbidities, such as ruminating or catastrophizing thoughts. Although research on combining computerized therapy with TMS is limited, the combination is typically proven effective in treating cognitive conditions; in our experience, patients are accepting of these applications and, upon completion, report the programs as helpful. Furthermore, the successful implementation of these programs can bolster patients' skill sets, empowering them to pursue continued mental health treatment, such as individual face-to-face therapy, following the completion of TMS.

Many brief psychotherapeutic skills can be taught or reinforced by the TMS technician during treatment sessions. Table 5–5 lists strategies that can be implemented while the patient is in the treatment session. For example, negative thinking about oneself, others, and one's future (Beck's negative triad; Beck et al. 1987) is pervasive in depression; learning to identify the triggers for one's negative thinking, maladaptive thought patterns, and typical cognitive errors can be easily accomplished with some basic training and reinforcement from the TMS technician. Acquisition of this type of skill is a neurobehavioral intervention with specific functional impact on the DLPFC, which correlates with improved functioning and "top-down" control of the limbic system (Ritchey et al. 2011).

Other behavioral skills that can be taught to depressed patients include brief mindfulness exercises, such as breathing mindfulness and a body scan (Kabat-Zinn 2013). Protocols lasting 10 and 20 minutes are readily available on several music streaming services and mobile applications. Meditation exercises are associated with greater top-down control in the short term and with downregulation of the limbic system over the long term ("bottom-up") (Chiesa et al. 2013). Having patients practice these skills while simultaneously receiving neuromodulation may facilitate faster acquisition, leading to a more durable antidepressant response. Research on such combinations is ongoing, but prospects appear promising and feasible to implement across TMS clinics.

Befriending is a treatment that increases social support for patients with depression, and NICE clinical guidelines suggest a role for this type of therapy for patients with chronic depression (Middleton et al. 2005). Befriending can be utilized during TMS to engage patients in an ongoing discussion of everyday topics and current events in a neutral, friendly, and nonconfrontational manner, without the expectation of solving problems or working through conflicts or emotions. Befriending is typically administered by unlicensed volunteers with 2–3 days of training (Mead et al. 2010). Harris et al. (1999) demonstrated the efficacy of befriending using volunteers for individuals with chronic depression. A meta-analysis of befriending therapy for depressive symptoms suggests the intervention has significant effects on depressive symptoms compared with usual care or no treatment (Mead et al. 2010). Befriending therapy has not been studied with TMS, but given its brief training period and application by unlicensed volunteers, it could be easily administered during treatment sessions.

Table 5–5. Brief "online" therapeutic activities for use during a transcranial magnetic stimulation therapy session

Goal setting

Positive imagery

Body scan mindfulness exercise

Mindfulness of the breath exercise

Progressive muscle relaxation

Psychoeducation about depression

Creating a sleep diary

Creating a nutrition diary

Breathing retraining to cope with anxiety

Identifying automatic thoughts and cognitive errors

Modifying negative thinking

Identifying triggers for depression

Activity scheduling

Psychoeducation regarding sleep

Psychoeducation regarding exercise

Creating symptom diaries

Leisure activities (e.g., listening to music or podcasts, watching TV)

Conclusion

The research supporting the combination of TMS with psychotherapy is still in its infancy. However, the importance of the combination of TMS with rehabilitative therapies, such as cognitive exercises, physical therapy, or occupational therapy, appears to be well documented for treating certain neurological disorders. We hypothesize that a patient's brain state matters while he or she is in the TMS treatment chair and that supporting treatment sessions with "online" therapeutic interventions may enhance outcomes. Furthermore, what a patient does with his or her time between TMS treatments ("offline") may also impact improvement. Thus, assessing a patient's psychotherapy history and prescribing psychotherapeutic activities is necessary when prescribing TMS for a patient with treatment-resistant depression.

KEY CLINICAL POINTS

- Patients prescribed TMS should be prescribed therapies delivered "offline" (i.e., therapies occurring over the course of TMS therapy but separately from the TMS treatment session). These include cognitive-behavioral therapy, behavioral activation, mindfulness-based cognitive-behavioral therapy, and interpersonal therapy.

- Patients prescribed TMS should be prescribed therapies delivered "online" (i.e., during the TMS treatment session). These include Internet-based therapies, mindfulness meditation, and befriending therapy.

- TMS technicians can provide brief therapeutic activities that do not require a licensed clinician and offer options to improve the use of patients' time in the treatment chair.

- Patients should be encouraged to engage in healthy behaviors, lifestyles, and relationships when prescribed TMS.

References

Beck AT, Rush AJ, Shaw BF, Emery G: Cognitive Therapy of Depression. New York, Guilford, 1987

Bajbouj M, Padberg F: A perfect match: noninvasive brain stimulation and psychotherapy. Eur Arch Psychiatry Clin Neurosci 264 (suppl 1):S27–S33, 2014 25253645

Biesheuvel-Leliefeld KEM, Kok GD, Bockting CLH, et al: Effectiveness of psychological interventions in preventing recurrence of depressive disorder: meta-analysis and meta-regression. J Affect Disord 174:400–410, 2015 25553400

Carpenter LL, Janicak PG, Aaronson ST, et al: Transcranial magnetic stimulation (TMS) for major depression: a multisite, naturalistic, observational study of acute treatment outcomes in clinical practice. Depress Anxiety 29(7):587–596, 2012 22689344

Chiesa A, Serretti A, Jakobsen JC: Mindfulness: top-down or bottom-up emotion regulation strategy? Clin Psychol Rev 33(1):82–96, 2013 23142788

Cuijpers P, Donker T, van Straten A, et al: Is guided self-help as effective as face-to-face psychotherapy for depression and anxiety disorders? A systematic review and meta-analysis of comparative outcome studies. Psychol Med 40(12):1943–1957, 2010 20406528

Cuijpers P, Donker T, Weissman MM, et al: Interpersonal psychotherapy for mental health problems: a comprehensive meta-analysis. Am J Psychiatry 173(7):680–687, 2016 27032627

Dimidjian S, Hollon SD, Dobson KS, et al: Randomized trial of behavioral activation, cognitive therapy, and antidepressant medication in the acute treatment of adults with major depression. J Consult Clin Psychol 74(4):658–670, 2006 16881773

Dobson KS, Hollon SD, Dimidjian S, et al: Randomized trial of behavioral activation, cognitive therapy, and antidepressant medication in the prevention of relapse and recurrence in major depression. J Consult Clin Psychol 76(3):468–477, 2008 18540740

Eisendrath SJ, Delucchi K, Bitner R, et al: Mindfulness-based cognitive therapy for treatment-resistant depression: a pilot study. Psychother Psychosom 77(5):319–320, 2008 18600038

Grassi G, Godini L, Grippo A, et al: Enhancing cognitive-behavioral therapy with repetitive transcranial magnetic stimulation in refractory obsessive-compulsive-disorder: a case report. Brain Stimulat 8(1):160–161, 2015 25456982

Guse B, Falkai P, Wobrock T: Cognitive effects of high-frequency repetitive transcranial magnetic stimulation: a systematic review. J Neural Transm (Vienna) 117(1):105–122, 2010 19859782

Harris T, Brown GW, Robinson R: Befriending as an intervention for chronic depression among women in an inner city, 1: randomised controlled trial. Br J Psychiatry 174:219–224 1999 10448446

Isserles M, Rosenberg O, Dannon P, et al: Cognitive-emotional reactivation during deep transcranial magnetic stimulation over the prefrontal cortex of depressive patients affects antidepressant outcome. J Affect Disord 128(3):235–242, 2011 20663568

Kabot-Zinn J: Full Castrophe Living: Using the Wisdom of Your Body and Mind to Face Stress, Pain, and Illness, 2nd Edition. New York, Bantam, 2013

Kakuda W, Abo M, Kaito N, et al: Six-day course of repetitive transcranial magnetic stimulation plus occupational therapy for post-stroke patients with upper limb hemiparesis: a case series study. Disabil Rehabil 32(10):801–807, 2010 20367405

Leong K, Chan P, Grabovac A, et al: Changes in mindfulness following repetitive transcranial magnetic stimulation for mood disorders. Can J Psychiatry 58(12):687–691, 2013 24331288

Marin M, Milad MR: Neuromodulation approaches for the treatment of post-traumatic stress disorder: stimulating the brain following exposure-based therapy. Curr Behav Neurosci Rep 2(2):67–71, 2015

Mead N, Lester H, Chew-Graham C, et al: Effects of befriending on depressive symptoms and distress: systematic review and meta-analysis. Br J Psychiatry 196(2):96–101, 2010 20118451

Middleton H, Shaw I, Hull S, Feder G: NICE guidelines for the management of depression. BMJ 330(7486):267–268 2005 15695252

Neacsiu AD: Neuromodulation Enhanced Cognitive Restructuring: A Proof of Concept Study. October 8, 2015. Available at: https://clinicaltrials.gov/ct2/show/NCT02573246. Accessed July 31, 2017.

Ochsner KN, Bunge SA, Gross JJ, et al: Rethinking feelings: an FMRI study of the cognitive regulation of emotion. J Cogn Neurosci 14(8):1215–1229, 2002 12495527

Osuch EA, Benson BE, Luckenbaugh DA, et al: Repetitive TMS combined with exposure therapy for PTSD: a preliminary study. J Anxiety Disord 23(1):54–59, 2009 18455908

Rabey JM, Dobronevsky E, Aichenbaum S, et al: Repetitive transcranial magnetic stimulation combined with cognitive training is a safe and effective modality for the treatment of Alzheimer's disease: a randomized, double-blind study. J Neural Transm (Vienna) 120(5):813–819, 2013 23076723

Ritchey M, Dolcos F, Eddington KM, et al: Neural correlates of emotional processing in depression: changes with cognitive behavioral therapy and predictors of treatment response. J Psychiatr Res 45(5):577–587, 2011 20934190

Rush AJ, Trivedi MH, Wisniewski SR, et al: Acute and longer-term outcomes in depressed outpatients requiring one or several treatment steps: a STAR*D report. Am J Psychiatry 163(11):1905–1917, 2006 17074942

Serafini G, Pompili M, Belvederi Murri M, et al: The effects of repetitive transcranial magnetic stimulation on cognitive performance in treatment-resistant depression: a systematic review. Neuropsychobiology 71(3):125–139, 2015 25925699

Strunk D: Depression. 2017. Available at: http://www.div12.org/psychological-treatments/disorders/depression/. Accessed April 4, 2017.

Teasdale JD, Segal ZV, Williams JMG, et al: Prevention of relapse/recurrence in major depression by mindfulness-based cognitive therapy. J Consult Clin Psychol 68(4):615–623, 2000 10965637

Vedeniapin A, Cheng L, George MS: Feasibility of simultaneous cognitive behavioral therapy and left prefrontal rTMS for treatment resistant depression. Brain Stimulat 3(4):207–210, 2010 20965449

Watts S, Mackenzie A, Thomas C, et al: CBT for depression: a pilot RCT comparing mobile phone vs. computer. BMC Psychiatry 13(1):49, 2013 23391304

Wiles N, Thomas L, Abel A, et al: Cognitive behavioural therapy as an adjunct to pharmacotherapy for primary care based patients with treatment resistant depression: results of the CoBalT randomised controlled trial. Lancet 381(9864):375–384, 2013 23219570

Williams M, Teasdale J, Segal Z, Kabot-Zinn J: The Mindful Way Through Depression: Freeing Yourself From Chronic Unhappiness. New York, Guilford, 2007

Yoon TH, Han SJ, Yoon TS, et al: Therapeutic effect of repetitive magnetic stimulation combined with speech and language therapy in post-stroke nonfluent aphasia. NeuroRehabilitation 36(1):107–114, 2015 25547773

Zheng CJ, Liao WJ, Xia WG: Effect of combined low-frequency repetitive transcranial magnetic stimulation and virtual reality training on upper limb function in subacute stroke: a double-blind randomized controlled trail. J Huazhong Univ Sci Technolog Med Sci 35(2):248–254, 2015 25877360

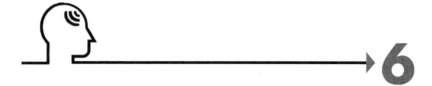

Managing Patients After Transcranial Magnetic Stimulation

How to Best Maintain Response and Remission

David L. Dunner, M.D., FACPsych
Richard A. Bermudes, M.D.

In this chapter, we review how to best manage patients who respond to transcranial magnetic stimulation (TMS) therapy. We focus on managing patients who receive TMS for major depression, but we also highlight key clinical points that can be applied to the management of bipolar disorder. Pivotal long-term studies with outcomes at 6 and 12 months post-

TMS will be reviewed. We make recommendations for clinical practice, keeping in mind the limitations of the existing database.

Difficulty of Achieving Sustained Remission With Treatment-Resistant Depression

Phases in the management of a depressive episode involve acute, continuation, and maintenance treatments (Frank et al. 1991). This perspective is important when using antidepressant pharmacotherapy and psychotherapy for individuals presenting for initial treatment or for chronic depression. The usual time frame allocated for *acute treatment* is 6–12 weeks to achieve a response or remission of symptoms. Research studies demonstrate that *continuation treatment* with pharmacotherapy and/or psychotherapy for an additional several months (4–12 months) reduces the likelihood of relapse (Dobson et al. 2008; Dunner 2001; Gelenberg et al. 2003; Keller et al. 2000, 2007a, 2007b; Klein et al. 2004; Kocsis et al. 2003; Paykel et al. 1995). *Maintenance treatment* is the next step (i.e., beyond 4–12 months), and evidence supports the efficacy of maintenance treatment for individuals with recurrent and chronic forms of depression (Frank et al. 1990; Keller et al. 2007a; Klein et al. 2004).

Research studies demonstrate that individuals with chronic forms of depression are more difficult to treat than individuals with acute depressive episodes (Dunner 2001). Furthermore, the Sequenced Treatment Alternatives to Relieve Depression (STAR*D) study showed a decrease in the rate of antidepressant response with repeated treatment failures (Gaynes et al. 2009; Rush et al. 2006). For example, individuals who experience three failed treatment trials have a low (about 15%) rate of remission in the subsequent trial. These data are similar to the results of a 2-year study of "treatment as usual" for individuals who had experienced multiple failed antidepressant treatments (Dunner et al. 2006; George et al. 2005).

Although most depressed patients respond well to treatment with psychotherapy and/or antidepressant pharmacotherapy, those who do not respond can be considered to have *treatment-resistant depression* (TRD). Sustained remission for patients with TRD is difficult to achieve with currently available options. A patient who attains remission after one prior antidepressant treatment failure has a 40% chance of relapse over the next year, whereas a patient who has attained remission after three prior antidepressant treatment failures has a 65% chance of relapse (Warden et al. 2007). Table 6–1 displays data from the STAR*D study and shows how increasing treatment resistance predicts an increasing

Table 6–1. Acute-phase remission rates and continuation-phase relapse rates for patients with increasing treatment resistance

STAR*D level	Acute-phase remission rate (%)	Continuation-phase relapse rate (%)
Level 1	37	40
Level 2	31	55
Level 3	14	65
Level 4	13	71

Note. Level 1 = initial treatment; Level 2 = failure to remit with Level 1 treatment; Level 3 = failure to remit with Level 2 treatment; Level 4 = failure to remit with Level 3 treatment.
Source. Data from Warden et al. 2007.

chance of relapse. When patients do not respond to multiple medications, their prognosis for long-term remission decreases. One might say the "durability of response" to antidepressant medications decreases with more failed trials.

Studies indicate that electroconvulsive therapy (ECT) is the most effective acute antidepressant treatment; however, in community settings it is difficult to achieve sustained remission with ECT. In a prospective, naturalistic study involving 347 patients at seven hospitals, clinical outcomes immediately after ECT and over a 24-week follow-up period were examined in relation to patient characteristics and treatment variables (Prudic et al. 2004). Remission rates during the acute phase were documented in the range of 30%–45%, in contrast to the 70% rates observed in research studies. Likewise, the probability of relapse during the continuation phase was as high as 64%. Patients who did not achieve remission during the acute phase had a poorer prognosis; however, the chance of relapse was high for all patients.

CLINICAL VIGNETTE

A 53-year-old man with a 4-year history of major depression presented for follow-up with his general psychiatrist after completing 6 weeks of acute TMS therapy 1 month earlier. The patient reported that he was sleeping well and had returned to work. His 9-item Patient Health Questionnaire (PHQ-9) score was 6 (mild). The treatment report from the TMS center indicated that his PHQ-9 score was 18 (severe) at baseline and 4 (remission) at the end of the TMS taper. He was currently taking the medications fluoxetine and L-methylfolate and fish oil. His psychiatrist discontinued the patient's previously prescribed quetiapine used as an augmentation agent and encouraged close mood monitoring, with the PHQ-9 to be completed every 2 weeks. He also encouraged the patient to initiate a healthy balance of leisure and productive activities and prescribed cognitive restructuring homework from a free online tool, MoodGYM (https://moodgym.com.au). The patient's follow-up appointment was set for 6 weeks later, but he was encouraged to call sooner if his symptoms worsened on the PHQ-9.

Durability of Antidepressant Response After Acute TMS

Once a patient responds to TMS, how long will the benefit last? Most patients pose this question during the consent process because they have experienced the disappointment of initially benefiting from an antidepressant treatment only to have their symptoms recur in the ensuing months. To investigate the mean remission time and the predictors associated with the treatment's duration, Cohen et al. (2009) performed a large retrospective, naturalistic study with 204 patients who underwent TMS therapy. Patients were followed for up to 6 months after acute treatment, and about 80% took psychotropic medications. The rate of event-free remission, with the end point defined as relapse (i.e., Hamilton Depression Rating Scale [HDRS] scores higher than 8), was 75.3% at 2 months, 60.0% at 3 months, 42.7% at 4 months, and 22.6% at 6 months. The mean duration of remission was approximately 4 months (119 days), with younger age and greater number of TMS sessions predicting greater durability of benefit.

Janicak et al. (2010) studied the durability of TMS in a population of 99 patients with major depressive disorder who had at least partially responded to acute TMS treatment while medication free. The patients then received antidepressant monotherapy for 24 weeks. If patients met predefined criteria for symptom worsening, they could receive TMS reintroduction (i.e., two sessions/week for 2 weeks and, if needed, five sessions/week for 4 additional weeks). Thirty-eight patients (38%) had symptom worsening and received TMS reintroduction. Thirty-two of the 38 patients (84%) benefited, with the mean time to reintroduction of TMS being 109 days and the mean number of TMS reintroduction sessions being 14.3. Fifteen patients needed more than one course of TMS, and five patients needed up to three courses. Ten patients relapsed despite access to flexible reintroduction of TMS. TMS was found to be a durable and safe treatment when patients were allowed "flexible reintroduction of TMS" combined with antidepressant monotherapy, and those who initially achieved remission had a better prognosis.

Dunner et al. (2014) reported the 1-year outcome in 257 patients with major depressive disorder treated with TMS. The acute treatment response was reported by Carpenter et al. (2012). Because this was an observational study conducted across 42 clinical practices in the United States, all patients were permitted clinician-directed treatment as usual (i.e., patients were not limited to a predefined single antidepressant as in the Janicak et al. [2010] study). Most were treated with antidepressant medications, and many received other medications (e.g., second-generation antipsychotic augmentation) during the acute and follow-up periods. Patients were allowed TMS reintroduction after acute treatment if deemed appropriate and prescribed by their physician. Other treatments such as psychotherapy were not reported. Over 60% of patients who had responded to or achieved remission during acute treatment with TMS sustained their response for 1 year. Ninety-three patients were treated with TMS during the ensuing 12 months of follow-up; the mean number of TMS sessions for this group was 16.2. Of the 45 subjects who did not maintain their remission or response status, 31 relapsed within 6 months. No safety or tolerability issues were noted during reintroduction of TMS.

These studies indicate that acute TMS therapy is beneficial for most patients with more chronic forms of depression for up to 4 months. Although research studies of TMS involved antidepressant medication–free patients, in clinical practice most patients continue medication after the acute phase and do not reduce their medication loads (Carpenter et al. 2012; Dunner et al. 2014). Having access to flexible doses of TMS to treat recurrent symptoms during the continuation phase improves durability, and most patients with such access require fewer TMS sessions to maintain their remission or response status. Continuing medication and reintroducing TMS is effective, but more research is needed to determine whether it is the optimal strategy for keeping patients well. For example, head-to-head studies comparing different protocols are needed, and researchers need to clarify whether participants are allowed to simultaneously receive other treatments with TMS.

Following TMS treatment, patients should be closely monitored, and their symptoms should be measured with a validated depression questionnaire. Research is needed to try to determine which patients are at most risk for relapse. Perhaps certain clinical or demographic variables predict relapse after TMS therapy. Several candidate variables were examined in the studies described in this section, but the results are inconsistent. Overall, patients who achieve remission with acute TMS have the best prognosis for maintaining response.

Maintenance TMS Sessions to Prevent Relapse or Recurrence

Because maintenance antidepressants and psychotherapy are effective in delaying a relapse or recurrence of depression, it would seem logical that providing TMS in some ongoing manner after response would also provide protection against relapse or recurrence. Table 6–2 summarizes several published TMS maintenance studies. Before 2015, the studies were retrospective or prospective observational studies without a comparison group, or they were case reports (Chatterjee et al. 2012; Demirtas-Tatlidede et al. 2008). Most defined maintenance TMS as scheduled sessions delivered weekly (e.g., 1–2 sessions/week) with a taper to a frequency of monthly (e.g., 1 session/month) delivered during the continuation phase. TMS delivered in this fashion preserves the response and remission rates obtained in the acute phase of treatment, or at least delays the decrement in the antidepressant effect achieved after the acute phase.

Two of the more recent studies used *deep TMS* (dTMS), which is a TMS device with an H1 coil rather than a figure-eight coil. These studies indicate that continuing TMS after acute response or remission can benefit patients. In the Harel et al. (2014) study, subjects participated in three distinct phases: 1) an acute phase for 4 weeks in which daily dTMS sessions were conducted five times per week, for a total of 20 sessions; 2) a first continuation treatment phase for 8 weeks, in which dTMS sessions were conducted twice a week for a total of 16 sessions; and 3) a second continuation treatment phase for 10 weeks, during which dTMS sessions were conducted once a week. Patients also continued their antidepressant medications. A significant decrease from baseline in HDRS score was found at the end of the acute phase ($P<0.0001$) and maintained throughout the 18-week study. Furthermore, the probability of response and remission increased over the course of the study, almost doubling for those who received continuation treatment.

The study by Levkovitz et al. (2015) also included a continuation treatment phase. The investigators randomly assigned 212 patients with TRD to monotherapy with dTMS or sham dTMS. Patients received daily sessions for 4 weeks, and 159 patients were available to continue twice-weekly sessions for 18 weeks. Response and remission rates were higher in the dTMS group than in the sham group ($P=0.013$ response; $P=0.005$ remission), and these benefits were preserved during the next 3 months with maintenance dTMS.

Research indicates that the benefits from TMS can be preserved with scheduled TMS sessions or with monitoring and then reintroducing TMS

Table 6–2. Maintenance studies of transcranial magnetic stimulation (TMS) for major depressive disorder

Study	Sample (*N*)	Design	Duration	Frequency of TMS	Outcome
O'Reardon et al. 2005	10	Retrospective	6 months to 6 years	1–2 sessions/week	3 patients maintained response
Connolly et al. 2012	42	Retrospective	6 months	Tapered to 1 session/month	62% maintained response
Fitzgerald et al. 2013	35	Prospective	1 year	Clustered 5 treatments over 2 days monthly	Delay in relapse
Richieri et al. 2013	59	Prospective	20 weeks	Tapered to 1 session/month	38% relapsed with maintenance, whereas 68% relapsed without maintenance
Harel et al. 2014	26	Prospective	18 weeks	Twice-weekly sessions for 8 weeks, then weekly	50% remission rate at end of study
Levkovitz et al. 2015	159	Prospective, sham controlled	12 weeks	Twice-weekly sessions	Active treatment superior to sham
Philip et al. 2016	49	Prospective, randomized	1 year	Monthly session	No significant differences between groups

Note. *N*=number of subjects.

when symptoms recur. A relevant concern is how to proceed clinically when patients are finishing their acute course. In a pilot study, Philip et al. (2016) attempted to address this issue by comparing outcomes in patients who received either scheduled TMS or observation after a 6-week course of TMS therapy. Forty-nine patients who met response criteria at the end of the acute phase were randomly assigned to one treatment monthly or to a monthly visit without TMS treatment during 12 months of follow-up. Patients in both groups who relapsed could receive reintroduction TMS. Importantly, subjects remained medication free during the acute and follow-up periods. Over 80% of subjects in both groups met criteria for remission at the end of acute treatment, defined as a score of 7 or less on the 17-item HDRS. Subsequently, there was no between-group difference in the number of patients who did not require TMS reintroduction (the primary outcome variable). However, TMS-treated patients had a slightly longer duration to first relapse (91 vs. 77 days); were slightly less likely to require retreatment with TMS (39% vs. 35%); required fewer retreatments in case of relapse (14.3 vs. 16.9); and showed a slightly higher percentage of response to retreatment (78% vs. 63%). In summary, in this study, which had a small sample size (i.e., 49), both approaches were comparable based on the primary and secondary outcomes.

Pharmacotherapy After Acute TMS Treatment to Prevent Relapse or Recurrence

Providers may choose to use antidepressant medication instead of TMS maintenance or reintroduction to prevent relapse. Schüle et al. (2003) reported a study of 26 medication-free patients with major depression who were treated with TMS, to which 39% responded after 2 weeks. Patients then received mirtazapine alone for 4 weeks, and then 13 of the patients had additional lithium, carbamazepine, or antipsychotic medication for the last 2 weeks. After 6 weeks, 77% achieved response. Although the authors suggested that pharmacotherapy after TMS could improve response rates, the sample size was small and the study duration was brief (i.e., within the time usually allocated for acute treatment).

Kedzior et al. (2015) performed a meta-analysis of 16 double-blind, parallel-design, randomized controlled trials utilizing acute TMS and reported the results of available follow-up data. Maintenance TMS was not provided in any of these trials, but medication after acute TMS treatment was allowed. Subjects received high-frequency TMS over the left

Table 6–3. Insurance coverage for maintenance transcranial magnetic stimulation (TMS)

Maintenance schedule	Typical coverage policies
Reintroduction TMS	Major plans will cover, but some conditions may apply. Most plans require at least a 50% improvement in depressive symptoms with TMS in a prior episode. Some plans require a 3- to 6-month waiting period.
Repeated courses of TMS treatment	Most plans will cover. Most require either a 50% improvement or remission in the previous course. Some plans require a 3- to 6-month waiting period.
Maintenance TMS	Typically, most plans do not cover "maintenance TMS." However, some plans may approve, on a case-by-case basis, time-limited scheduled TMS—that is, "extended taper"—with a plan to decrease utilization.

dorsolateral prefrontal cortex for 2–3 weeks (i.e., 10–15 treatment sessions). Most of the studies had brief follow-up data (i.e., 1–4 weeks after the last TMS session); only one study reported more than 3 months of follow-up. The authors noted that the durability of the antidepressant effect of TMS was "small but stable" and that posttreatment antidepressant pharmacotherapy tended to enhance the antidepressant effect. The analysis was limited, however, because of the relatively short courses of TMS therapy used in the 16 trials. By contrast, most patients today receive up to 6 weeks of treatment (30 sessions) during the acute course.

In clinical practice, providers advise patients to monitor their symptoms closely and continue with psychotherapy and pharmacotherapy after TMS. It is rare for insurance policies to include coverage of TMS during the continuation or maintenance phases (Table 6–3). We recommend that patients who have responded to TMS in the past restart TMS if they relapse, and most major insurance policies will cover "reintroduction treatment" on a limited basis. In certain communities and in specific clinical circumstances, however, patients are prescribed scheduled TMS treatments (McClintock et al. 2017; Perera et al. 2016). Patients with multiple relapses who continue to benefit from reintroduction may benefit from a more frequent schedule of TMS therapy (e.g., once a week) with a longer taper over many months, as is often the practice with ECT treatment (Sackeim 2016).

Psychotherapy After Acute TMS Treatment to Prevent Relapse or Recurrence

There is no research indicating that psychotherapy improves the durability of TMS. However, certain psychotherapies are effective for residual depressive symptoms and relapse prophylaxis (Dobson et al. 2008; Frank et al. 1991). For example, mindfulness-based cognitive therapy is effective for patients with TRD, especially those who have a history of childhood trauma (Williams et al. 2014), unstable pharmacotherapy remitters (Segal et al. 2010), and those who have experienced three or more depressive episodes (Piet and Hougaard 2011). Many TMS practitioners will refer patients to psychotherapy as the patients' depressive symptoms are decreasing and they are responding to TMS. Many patients report increased or new benefits from psychotherapy, and restarting psychotherapy can be an opportunity to work on recovery and correct maladaptive patterns that may have developed during their depressive illness. Other important lifestyle changes can be effective as the patient responds (e.g., dietary changes, weight loss, improved sleep hygiene, exercise) (see Chapter 5, "Transcranial Magnetic Stimulation and Psychotherapy").

CLINICAL VIGNETTE

The patient is a 27-year-old woman with a 3-year history of major depression. After 6 weeks of TMS therapy, her PHQ-9 score decreased from a baseline of 21 (severe) to a posttreatment of 9 (mild). During her TMS taper, she started duloxetine and began interpersonal psychotherapy. At her 1-month post-TMS visit, her PHQ-9 score was 12, so duloxetine was increased from 30 to 60 mg/day. She presented to her general psychiatrist for her second follow-up visit with a PHQ-9 score of 17 and reported worsening depressive symptoms since tapering TMS 3 months earlier, as well as sexual side effects from her antidepressant. Her general psychiatrist referred her for reintroduction TMS therapy, which the patient began with two sessions/week for 2 weeks, at which point her PHQ-9 score was 9. She then received one session/week for 3 weeks followed by one session every other week for 4 weeks (i.e., a total of nine sessions over 9 weeks). One month later at her next visit, her PHQ-9 score was 5.

Maintenance TMS After Response to ECT

There are a few reports of using TMS to maintain response to ECT. Brunelin et al. (2010) reported a patient diagnosed with bipolar I rapid cycling. This patient was treated with 191 ECT treatments over a 3-year period to prevent depressive relapses. However, she developed atrial fibrillation, and use of ECT was prohibited by her cardiologist. She was then treated with TMS during an acute depressive episode, and this was followed by a maintenance TMS program of two treatments on the same day every 2 weeks for a year. She exhibited no depressive relapses. She was also being treated with lithium carbonate.

Noda et al. (2013) reported the results of six patients (four with major depression and two with bipolar depression) who were successfully treated with ECT, which was followed with maintenance TMS once or twice weekly. Five of the patients were able to maintain their response over a 6- to 12-month follow-up.

Maintenance TMS for Bipolar Disorder

Very limited data are available on the durability of TMS for other depressive disorders or special populations (e.g., geriatric patients). The durability of the effect of TMS in patients with bipolar depression was reported by Dell'Osso et al. (2011). Eleven subjects with bipolar I and II disorder with TRD were treated with TMS. Six patients responded, including four who achieved remission; three patients showed a partial response, and two showed no response. Patients were treated with appropriate medications during TMS and thereafter and were followed for 1 year. Four of the responders maintained their response, and three of those in remission continued in remission. One of the responders and one of the patients who achieved remission experienced a depressive syndrome at 2-month follow-up. Two partial responders experienced depressive recurrences, and one partial responder achieved remission by the end of follow-up.

Li et al. (2004) reported on seven patients with bipolar depression who responded to acute treatment with TMS and were then treated with TMS weekly for up to 1 year. Three of the patients maintained a score of 13 or lower on the HDRS for up to 1 year of follow-up. The remaining four patients experienced multiple relapses and did not complete the study. Patients were also receiving various psychotropic medications during the study.

Safety and Tolerability of Maintenance TMS

TMS is safe and tolerable outside of the typical course of 4–6 weeks of treatment. In the 12-month study conducted by Philip et al. (2016), there were no serious device-related adverse events reported, including hospitalizations, suicide attempts, and seizures. Janicak et al. (2010) reported that about 5% of patients had device-related adverse effects, such as application site pain, headaches, and muscle twitching, during 6 months of follow-up. Most patients acclimate to TMS quite rapidly after a previous course and typically have no adverse effects or serious reactions to extended courses.

Conclusion

TMS therapy has a durable antidepressant effect for patients with treatment-resistant depression when used as monotherapy. This durability is enhanced when other treatments or reintroduction TMS is used during the continuation phase of treatment. How best to optimize the durability of TMS is still unclear. It is unknown whether different stimulation protocols are more durable than others, because most of the studies have involved high-frequency stimulation over the left dorsolateral prefrontal cortex. Furthermore, most of the studies conducted beyond 90 days have used TMS systems with figure-eight coils rather than dTMS. Utilizing TMS to enhance the duration of response to other treatments is not fully delineated, although there are some indications that TMS may enhance the duration of response to medication and ECT (Noda et al. 2013).

It is not clear from the literature to date whether there is a uniform treatment package that should be prescribed for each patient who responds to or who achieves remission during TMS. Figure 6–1 provides several options for patients that may improve the durability of response or remission. Prescribers should consider a patient-centered approach that takes into account the individual's history of treatment response, the number and severity of depressive episodes, and access to studied treatments. Patients with treatment-resistant depression who have responded to TMS should be managed with a combination of pharmacotherapy, psychotherapy, and TMS, with the goal of increasing the number of days spent in remission.

KEY CLINICAL POINTS

- TMS is a safe and effective treatment for individuals with treatment-resistant depression, and this benefit persists for at least 1 year in some patients.

- Patients completing TMS should have their moods assessed with a validated instrument at regular intervals for early identification of symptom recurrence.

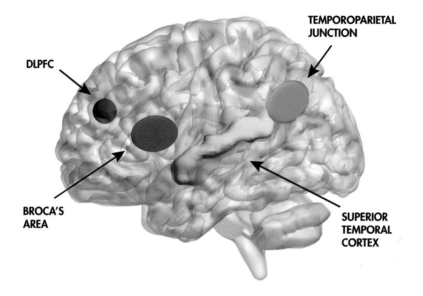

Plate 1. (*Figure 9–1*) Schizophrenia circuit.

Left-sided lateral view of the brain outlining regions of interest in schizophrenia. The auditory and linguistic areas of the brain responsible for speech, including the right and left superior temporal cortex, Broca's area, and the left temporoparietal area, are implicated in auditory hallucinations. The negative symptoms of schizophrenia are associated with hypoactivity of the dorsolateral prefrontal cortex (DLPFC). Image was visualized with the BrainNet Viewer (Xia et al. 2013).

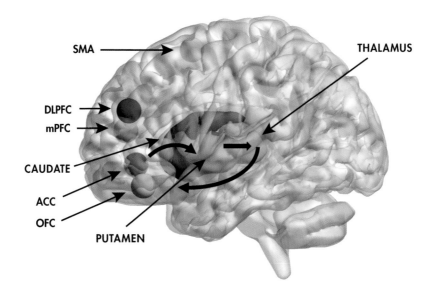

Plate 2. *(Figure 9–2)* Obsessive-compulsive disorder (OCD) circuit.

Left-sided lateral view of the brain with medial structures also visible. Evidence suggests that the orbitofronto-striato-pallido-thalamic circuit underlies the core symptoms of OCD. This well-defined circuitry involves the dorsolateral prefrontal cortex (DLPFC), orbitofrontal cortex (OFC), medial prefrontal cortex (mPFC), anterior cingulate cortex (ACC), supplementary motor area (SMA), and basal ganglia, composed of the caudate and putamen (Del Casale et al. 2011). Image was visualized with the BrainNet Viewer (Xia et al. 2013).

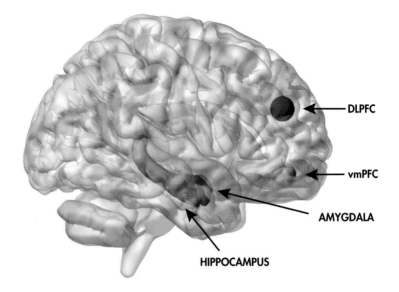

Plate 3. *(Figure 9–3)* Posttraumatic stress disorder (PTSD) circuit.

Right-sided lateral view of structures implicated in PTSD. Functional neuroimaging findings in PTSD support the hypothesis that the amygdala is hyperresponsive, and ventral portions of medial prefrontal cortex (vmPFC) and right dorsolateral prefrontal cortex are hyporesponsive. Hippocampal volume and function appear to be abnormal as well. Image was visualized with the BrainNet Viewer (Xia et al. 2013).

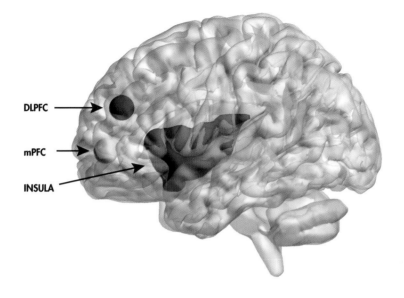

Plate 4. *(Figure 9–4)* Addiction circuit.

Left-sided lateral view of potential transcranial magnetic stimulation (TMS) targets for addiction therapy. Damage to the insula has been associated with an increased ability to stop smoking, whereas cue activation of the medial prefrontal cortex (mPFC) has been seen in alcoholic patients. The most common target to date is the left dorsolateral prefrontal cortex (DLPFC), where TMS may have a role in craving reduction. The DLPFC has been studied in patients for a variety of addictions, including nicotine, alcohol, recreational drugs, and food. Image was visualized with the BrainNet Viewer (Xia et al. 2013*).

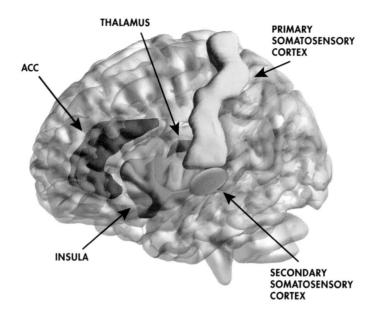

Plate 5. *(Figure 9–5)* Pain circuit.

Left-sided view of both lateral and medial structures involved in chronic pain. Pain processing is complex; however, a general conceptual framework has been adopted in which the structures involved are divided into lateral and medial components, which contribute to the sensory-discriminative and affective-motivational dimensions of pain, respectively. The lateral system includes the primary and secondary somatosensory cortices, whereas the insula and anterior cingulate cortex (ACC) are the main targets of the medial system. The thalamus plays a processing role in both systems. Image was visualized with the BrainNet Viewer (Xia et al. 2013).

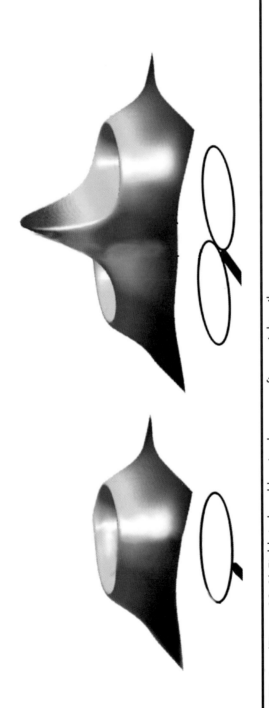

PLATE 6. *(Figure 10–1)* Fields induced by circular versus figure-eight coils.

Electric field intensity is displayed by both height and color.
Source. Based on Cohen et al. 1990 and Thielscher and Kammer 2002.

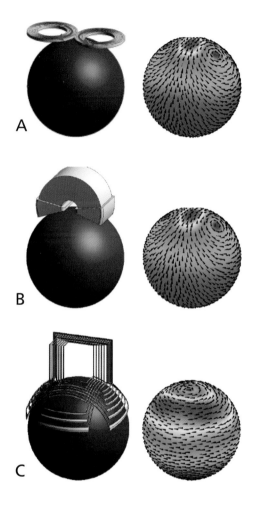

Plate 7. *(Figure 10–2)* Electric fields from three example coil designs.

(A) Figure-eight coil, air core; (B) figure-eight coil, ferromagnetic core; and (C) H1 coil, air core.

Souce. Adapted from Deng et al. 2013.

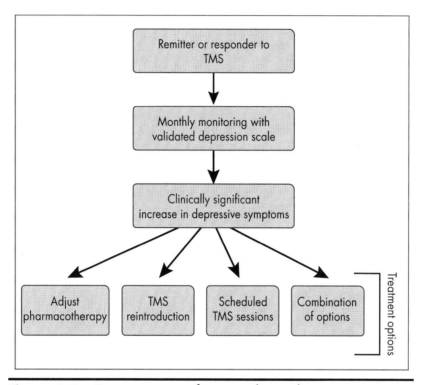

Figure 6–1. Treatment options for responders and remitters to optimize durability of transcranial magnetic stimulation (TMS).

- Maintenance pharmacotherapy and psychotherapy are effective strategies to treat residual depressive symptoms and prevent relapse.
- Flexible access to TMS for symptom recurrence is an effective strategy for helping patients maintain the acute benefits of TMS therapy.

References

Brunelin J, Ben Maklouf W, Nicolas A, et al: Successful switch to maintenance rTMS after maintenance ECT in refractory bipolar disorder. Brain Stimul 3(4):238–239, 2010 20965454

Carpenter LL, Janicak PG, Aaronson ST, et al: Transcranial magnetic stimulation (TMS) for major depression: a multisite, naturalistic, observational study of acute treatment outcomes in clinical practice. Depress Anxiety 29(7):587–596, 2012 22689344

Chatterjee B, Kumar N, Jha S: Role of repetitive transcranial magnetic stimulation in maintenance treatment of resistant depression. Indian J Psychol Med 34(3):286–289, 2012 23440309

Cohen RB, Boggio PS, Fregni F: Risk factors for relapse after remission with repetitive transcranial magnetic stimulation for the treatment of depression. Depress Anxiety 26(7):682–688, 2009 19170101

Connolly KR, Helmer A, Cristancho MA, et al: Effectiveness of transcranial magnetic stimulation in clinical practice post-FDA approval in the United States: results observed with the first 100 consecutive cases of depression at an academic medical center. J Clin Psychiatry 73(4):e567–e573, 2012 22579164

Dell'Osso B, D'Urso N, Castellano F, et al: Long-term efficacy after acute augmentative repetitive transcranial magnetic stimulation in bipolar depression: a 1-year follow-up study. J ECT 27(2):141–144, 2011 20966770

Demirtas-Tatlidede A, Mechanic-Hamilton D, Press DZ, et al: An open-label, prospective study of repetitive transcranial magnetic stimulation (rTMS) in the long-term treatment of refractory depression: reproducibility and duration of the antidepressant effect in medication-free patients. J Clin Psychiatry 69(6):930–934, 2008 18505308

Dobson KS, Hollon SD, Dimidjian S, et al: Randomized trial of behavioral activation, cognitive therapy, and antidepressant medication in the prevention of relapse and recurrence in major depression. J Consult Clin Psychol 76(3):468–477, 2008 18540740

Dunner DL: Acute and maintenance treatment of chronic depression. J Clin Psychiatry 62 (suppl 6):10–16, 2001 11310814

Dunner DL, Rush AJ, Russell JM, et al: Prospective, long-term, multicenter study of the naturalistic outcomes of patients with treatment-resistant depression. J Clin Psychiatry 67(5):688–695, 2006 16841617

Dunner DL, Aaronson ST, Sackeim HA, et al: A multisite, naturalistic, observational study of transcranial magnetic stimulation for patients with pharmacoresistant major depressive disorder: durability of benefit over a 1-year follow-up period. J Clin Psychiatry 75(12):1394–1401, 2014 25271871

Fitzgerald PB, Grace N, Hoy KE, et al: An open label trial of clustered maintenance rTMS for patients with refractory depression. Brain Stimul 6(3):292–297, 2013 22683273

Frank E, Kupfer DJ, Perel JM, et al: Three-year outcomes for maintenance therapies in recurrent depression. Arch Gen Psychiatry 47(12):1093–1099, 1990 2244793

Frank E, Prien RF, Jarrett RB, et al: Conceptualization and rationale for consensus definitions of terms in major depressive disorder: remission, recovery, relapse, and recurrence. Arch Gen Psychiatry 48(9):851–855, 1991 1929776

Gaynes BN, Warden D, Trivedi MH, et al: What did STAR*D teach us? Results from a large-scale, practical, clinical trial for patients with depression. Psychiatr Serv 60(11):1439–1445, 2009 19880458

Gelenberg AJ, Trivedi MH, Rush AJ, et al: Randomized, placebo-controlled trial of nefazodone maintenance treatment in preventing recurrence in chronic depression. Biol Psychiatry 54(8):806–817, 2003 14550680

George MS, Rush AJ, Marangell LB, et al: A one-year comparison of vagus nerve stimulation with treatment as usual for treatment-resistant depression. Biol Psychiatry 58(5):364–373, 2005 16139582

Harel EV, Rabany L, Deutsch L, et al: H-coil repetitive transcranial magnetic stimulation for treatment resistant major depressive disorder: an 18-week continuation safety and feasibility study. World J Biol Psychiatry 15(4):298–306, 2014 22313023

Janicak PG, Nahas Z, Lisanby SH, et al: Durability of clinical benefit with transcranial magnetic stimulation (TMS) in the treatment of pharmacoresistant major depression: assessment of relapse during a 6-month, multisite, open-label study. Brain Stimul 3(4):187–199, 2010 20965447

Kedzior KK, Reitz SK, Azorina V, et al: Durability of the antidepressant effect of the high-frequency repetitive transcranial magnetic stimulation (rTMS) in the absence of maintenance treatment in major depression: a systematic review and meta-analysis of 16 double-blind, randomized, sham-controlled trials. Depress Anxiety 32(3):193–203, 2015 25683231

Keller MB, McCullough JP, Klein DN, et al: A comparison of nefazodone, the cognitive behavioral-analysis system of psychotherapy, and their combination for the treatment of chronic depression. N Engl J Med 342(20):1462–1470, 2000 10816183

Keller MB, Trivedi MH, Thase ME, et al: The Prevention of Recurrent Episodes of Depression With Venlafaxine for Two Years (PREVENT) study: outcomes from the 2-year and combined maintenance phases. J Clin Psychiatry 68(8):1246–1256, 2007a 17854250

Keller MB, Trivedi MH, Thase ME, et al: The Prevention of Recurrent Episodes of Depression With Venlafaxine for Two Years (PREVENT) study: outcomes from the acute and continuation phases. Biol Psychiatry 62(12):1371–1379, 2007b 17825800

Klein DN, Santiago NJ, Vivian D, et al: Cognitive-behavioral analysis system of psychotherapy as a maintenance treatment for chronic depression. J Consult Clin Psychol 72(4):681–688, 2004 15301653

Kocsis JH, Rush AJ, Markowitz JC, et al: Continuation treatment of chronic depression: a comparison of nefazodone, cognitive behavioral analysis system of psychotherapy, and their combination. Psychopharmacol Bull 37(4):73–87, 2003 15131518

Levkovitz Y, Isserles M, Padberg F, et al: Efficacy and safety of deep transcranial magnetic stimulation for major depression: a prospective multicenter randomized controlled trial. World Psychiatry 14(1):64–73, 2015 25655160

Li X, Nahas Z, Anderson B, et al: Can left prefrontal rTMS be used as a maintenance treatment for bipolar depression? Depress Anxiety 20(2):98–100, 2004 15390210

McClintock SM, Reti IM, Carpenter LL, et al: Consensus recommendations for the clinical application of repetitive transcranial magnetic stimulation (rTMS) in the treatment of depression. Clin Psychiatry May 23, 2017 [Epub ahead of print]

Noda Y, Daskalakis ZJ, Ramos C, et al: Repetitive transcranial magnetic stimulation to maintain treatment response to electroconvulsive therapy in depression: a case series. Front Psychiatry 4:73, 2013 23888145

O'Reardon JP, Blumner KH, Peshek AD, et al: Long-term maintenance therapy for major depressive disorder with rTMS. J Clin Psychiatry 66(12):1524–1528, 2005 16401152

Paykel ES, Ramana R, Cooper Z, et al: Residual symptoms after partial remission: an important outcome in depression. Psychol Med 25(6):1171–1180, 1995 8637947

Perera T, George MS, Grammer G, et al: The Clinical TMS Society consensus review and treatment recommendations for TMS therapy for major depressive disorder. Brain Stimul 9(3):336–346 2016 27090022

Philip NS, Dunner DL, Dowd SM, et al: Can medication free, treatment-resistant depressed patients who initially respond to TMS be maintained off medications? A prospective, 12-month multisite randomized pilot study. Brain Stimul 9(2):251–257, 2016 26708778

Piet J, Hougaard E: The effect of mindfulness-based cognitive therapy for prevention of relapse in recurrent major depressive disorder: a systematic review and meta-analysis. Clin Psychol Rev 31(6):1032–1040, 2011 21802618

Prudic J, Olfson M, Marcus SC, et al: Effectiveness of electroconvulsive therapy in community settings. Biol Psychiatry 55(3):301–312, 2004 14744473

Richieri R, Guedj E, Michel P, et al: Maintenance transcranial magnetic stimulation reduces depression relapse: a propensity-adjusted analysis. J Affect Disord 151(1):129–135, 2013 23790811

Rush AJ, Trivedi MH, Wisniewski SR, et al: Acute and longer-term outcomes in depressed outpatients requiring one or several treatment steps: a STAR*D report. Am J Psychiatry 163(11):1905–1917, 2006 17074942

Sackeim HA: Acute continuation and maintenance treatment of major depressive episodes with transcranial magnetic stimulation. Brain Stimul 9(3):313–319, 2016 27052475

Schüle C, Zwanzger P, Baghai T, et al: Effects of antidepressant pharmacotherapy after repetitive transcranial magnetic stimulation in major depression: an open follow-up study. J Psychiatr Res 37(2):145–153, 2003 12842168

Segal ZV, Bieling P, Young T, et al: Antidepressant monotherapy vs sequential pharmacotherapy and mindfulness-based cognitive therapy, or placebo, for relapse prophylaxis in recurrent depression. Arch Gen Psychiatry 67(12):1256–1264, 2010 21135325

Warden D, Rush AJ, Trivedi MH, et al: The STAR*D project results: a comprehensive review of findings. Curr Psychiatry Rep 9(6):449–459, 2007 18221624

Williams JM, Crane C, Barnhofer T, et al: Mindfulness-based cognitive therapy for preventing relapse in recurrent depression: a randomized dismantling trial. J Consult Clin Psychol 82(2):275–286, 2014 24294837

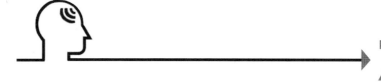

Transcranial Magnetic Stimulation and Other Neuromodulation Therapies

Karl I. Lanocha, M.D.
Philip G. Janicak, M.D.

Neuromodulation describes any treatment that modifies or alters the activity of the nervous system. In the broadest sense, this term could be said to refer to pharmaceuticals, but the term generally is used to refer to treatments that use some form of electromagnetic stimulus. Advances in therapeutic neuromodulation now provide clinicians with various options beyond medication and psychotherapy to treat depression.

Although electroconvulsive therapy (ECT) is the prototype therapeutic neuromodulation approach, many patients with treatment-resistant depression are not appropriate candidates or are unwilling to consider ECT because of its disadvantages. More recent alternatives provide a wide range of approaches, for example, transcranial magnetic stimulation (TMS) and vagus nerve stimulation (VNS), both of which have U.S. Food and Drug Administration (FDA) indications for management of more difficult-to-treat depressions. Other approaches, none of which has FDA clearance yet, include focal electrically administered seizure therapy (FEAST), magnetic seizure therapy (MST), deep brain stimulation (DBS), and transcranial direct current stimulation (tDCS). These approaches can be categorized based on the need for a surgical procedure (i.e., invasive vs. noninvasive) and the need to produce a seizure to achieve their clinical benefit (i.e., convulsive vs. nonconvulsive) (Table 7–1). In this chapter, we focus on the potential role of TMS relative to ECT. We provide a broad overview of the literature and make recommendations for patient selection. A full discussion of other emerging techniques is beyond the scope of this chapter, but brief descriptions are included at the end of the chapter to provide a broader context for understanding TMS.

TMS and ECT for Management of Depression

TMS is often compared with ECT. Although both treatments are forms of neuromodulation, they use very different technologies and methods of administration. ECT involves direct application of an electrical current via electrodes, whereas TMS uses a magnetic field to induce an electrical field without the use of electrodes. ECT stimulates the entire brain, from cortex to brain stem, whereas TMS stimulates only a small, localized area of the cortex. Because the therapeutic element of ECT is a generalized seizure, it must be modified by the use of anesthesia and neuromuscular blockade. TMS is nonconvulsive and noninvasive and is administered while a person is fully awake and is completely independent throughout the treatment course. This accounts for the very different risk and side-effect profiles of ECT and TMS, particularly effects on cognition.

Studies have considered TMS as a potential acute treatment alternative to ECT; the use of TMS as an acute complementary strategy with ECT; the durability of clinical effect for TMS versus ECT; the role of TMS as a maintenance strategy after a successful acute course of ECT; the relative cost-effectiveness of TMS and ECT; and patient preference for TMS versus ECT. These topics are discussed in the following subsections.

Table 7–1. Comparison of different forms of neuromodulation

	Seizure	**No seizure**
Noninvasive	Electroconvulsive therapy (ECT)[a]	Transcranial magnetic stimulation (TMS)[a]
	Magnetic seizure therapy (MST)	Cranial electrotherapy stimulation (CES)
	Focal electrically administered seizure therapy (FEAST)	Transcranial direct current stimulation (tDCS)
		External trigeminal nerve stimulation
		Transcutaneous auricular vagus nerve stimulation (taVNS)
Invasive		Deep brain stimulation (DBS)[b]
		Vagus nerve stimulation (VNS)[a]
		Epidural prefrontal cortical stimulation (EpCS)

Note. Invasive is defined as requiring a surgical procedure.
[a]Procedure has been cleared by the U.S. Food and Drug Administration for depression.
[b]Procedure has been cleared by the U.S. Food and Drug Administration for Parkinson's disease and OCD.

TMS Versus ECT for Acute Treatment

Ten published studies directly compare TMS and ECT for patients with a major depressive episode deemed appropriate for ECT. Participants in these studies suffered primarily from unipolar depression, although some also had bipolar depression. All but two of the studies involved random assignment to either treatment, all but one used left-sided high-frequency TMS, and four used single-blind assessments. The studies varied in regard to the type of ECT and TMS devices, ECT electrode placement (i.e., bilateral, unilateral nondominant, unilateral nondominant switched to bilateral), and the number of sessions with either treatment approach. With these limitations in mind, the results of these studies are summarized as follows: five left-sided high-frequency trials (four randomized and one open) showed antidepressant equivalence between the two therapies; four left-sided high-frequency trials (three randomized and one open) showed superiority for ECT over TMS; and one right-sided low-frequency trial showed superiority for ECT over TMS. Of note, *no trial results showed superiority for TMS over ECT*. All trials, however, demonstrated either comparable or better tolerability with TMS, particularly regarding cognitive effects (e.g., Martis et al. 2003). Furthermore, by present standards, no trial provided an optimal course of TMS. Table 7–2 summarizes these trials in more detail. Despite methodological shortcomings, the studies provide preliminary guidance about the relative advantages and disadvantages of both approaches.

In addition, three meta-analyses consider the acute benefit of TMS compared with ECT. The first meta-analysis (Micallef-Trigona 2014) considered nine trials (N=384) that met the author's criteria for inclusion. Patients were randomly assigned to either treatment and assessed with the Hamilton Depression Rating Scale (HDRS). Although both treatment arms produced a significant decrease from baseline scores, ECT was superior to TMS in terms of total point reduction (i.e., 15.4 vs. 9.3, respectively; $P<0.01$). The second meta-analysis (Ren et al. 2014) considered nine trials (N=425). On the basis of HDRS change scores, ECT was superior to TMS in terms of response ($P<0.03$) and remission ($P<0.01$). When patients with psychotic symptoms were excluded, however, response and remission rates did not differ between the two groups. A third meta-analysis (Xie et al. 2013) considered nine trials (N=395). The authors reported that differing parameters significantly altered the response to TMS and suggested that this issue should be addressed in future studies that compare TMS with ECT.

TMS COMBINED WITH ECT FOR ACUTE TREATMENT

In a published pilot study, Pridmore (2000) compared unilateral nondominant ECT (UND ECT) with UND ECT plus TMS. Over the 2-week trial, one group (n=11) received UND ECT three times per week, and the second group (n=11) received one UND ECT session followed by four daily TMS sessions. Both groups experienced a comparable response, but the UND ECT plus TMS group experienced fewer adverse events.

TMS VERSUS ECT: DURABILITY OF CLINICAL EFFECT

Two of the acute trials described in Table 7–2 also reported their patients' clinical status after 6 months. Dannon et al. (2002) found no differences in the relapse rates (i.e., 20%) based on the HDRS-17 and the Global Assessment of Functioning (GAF) Scale in either the ECT (N=20) or TMS (N=21) groups. Eranti et al. (2007) also reported no difference between the ECT (N=22) and TMS (N=24) groups based on the HDRS-17 change

Table 7–2. Comparative studies of transcranial magnetic stimulation (TMS) and electroconvulsive therapy (ECT)

	Outcome		Comments[a]
	ECT (%)	TMS (%)	
Left-sided high-frequency TMS vs. ECT: acute randomized trials			
Grunhaus et al. 2000	16/20 (80%)	9/20 (45%)	Response rate: HDRS-17 ($\geq$50%); GAS ($\geq$60) Unblinded assessments TMS comparable to UND/BL ECT in nonpsychotic major depression; up to 20 treatments
Pridmore et al. 2000	11/16 (69%)	11/16 (69%)	Remission rate: HDRS-17 ($\geq$8) Single-blind assessments UND ECT (mean=10.5 treatments); TMS (20 treatments)
Janicak et al. 2002, 2005	6/14 (43%)	7/17 (41%)	Response rate: HDRS-24 ($\geq$50%; $\geq$8) Unblinded assessments 2–4 weeks of treatment; BL ECT
Grunhaus et al. 2003	12/20 (60%) 6/20 (30%)	11/20 (55%) 6/20 (30%)	Response rate: HDRS-17 ($\geq$50%; <10); GAS ($\geq$60) Remission rate: HDRS-17 ($\leq$8) Single-blind assessments UND ECT (mean=10.5 treatments); TMS (20 treatments)
Rosa et al. 2006	6/15 (40%)	10/20 (50%)	Response rate: HDRS-17 ($\geq$50%) Single-blind assessments UND/BL ECT (up to 4 weeks); TMS (20 treatments)

Table 7–2. Comparative studies of transcranial magnetic stimulation (TMS) and electroconvulsive therapy (ECT) *(continued)*

	Outcome		Comments[a]
	ECT (%)	TMS (%)	
Left-sided high-frequency TMS vs. ECT: acute randomized trials *(continued)*			
Eranti et al. 2007	13/22 (59%)	4/24 (17%)	Remission rate: HDRS-17 (≤8) Single-blind assessments UND/BL ECT (mean=6.3 treatments); TMS (mean=13.7 treatments)
Keshtkar et al. 2011	68% improvement from baseline (n=40)	29% improvement from baseline (n=33)	HDRS-21 Unblinded assessments BL ECT (10 treatments); TMS (10 treatments)
Left-sided high-frequency TMS vs. ECT: acute open trials			
O'Connor et al. 2003	62% mean improvement from baseline (n=14)	10% mean improvement from baseline (n=14)	HDRS-17 Unblinded assessments UND ECT (6–12 treatments); TMS (10 treatments)
Schulze-Rauschenbach et al. 2005	6/14 (43%)	7/16 (44%)	Response rate: HDRS-17 (≥50%) Unblinded assessments UND ECT (mean=10 treatments); TMS (mean=10 treatments)

Table 7–2. Comparative studies of transcranial magnetic stimulation (TMS) and electroconvulsive therapy (ECT) *(continued)*

	Outcome		
	ECT (%)	**TMS (%)**	**Comments**[a]
Right-sided low-frequency TMS vs. ECT: acute randomized trial			
Hansen et al. 2011	26% higher rate of partial remission with ECT vs. TMS (*P*<0.04)	TMS (*n*=30) ECT (*n*=30)	HDRS-17 Unblinded assessments UND ECT (9 treatments); TMS (15 treatments)

Note. BL ECT=bilateral ECT; GAS=Global Assessment Scale; HDRS=Hamilton Depression Rating Scale (17-item or 24-item version); UND/BL ECT=unilateral nondominant ECT switched to bilateral ECT; UND ECT=unilateral nondominant ECT.
[a]For response and remission rates, values within parentheses indicate criteria defining response.

scores. A more recent, large retrospective study considered 300 patients with recurrent major depression, half of whom received a course of TMS and half of whom received a course of ECT (Jin et al. 2016). Jin et al. reported that although the acute response rate was greater in the ECT group than in the TMS group (i.e., 58.7% vs. 46.0%; $P<0.05$), the survival rate was comparable between groups.

TMS FOR MAINTENANCE TREATMENT AFTER ACUTE ECT RESPONSE

Given the high rates of relapse after an acute response to ECT, there is a need to develop effective maintenance strategies; Jelovac et al. (2013) provide an overview of current evidence with respect to relapse after acute ECT. Studies in adult and geriatric patients employed maintenance medication, ECT, or their combination and yielded mixed results (Kellner et al. 2006, 2016). Thus, no clear guidance is yet available on how to provide an optimally effective approach.

Two case series have considered the relative long-term benefits of TMS as one such strategy for maintaining ECT benefit. The first case series included six patients (four with unipolar and two with bipolar depression) who were followed for 6–13 months and received once- or twice-weekly bilateral TMS maintenance treatments after a successful acute course of ECT (Noda et al. 2013). The authors reported that five of the six patients were able to maintain their response status during this time period, as supported by change in scores on the Quick Inventory of Depressive Symptomatology—Self-Report (QIDS-SR). In the second case series, six patients (five of whom had major depression) were transitioned from maintenance ECT to maintenance TMS (administered on average every 3.5 weeks) because of adverse events or patient preference (Cristancho et al. 2013). As demonstrated by change in scores on the Beck Depression Inventory (BDI) from the initiation of TMS therapy, all patients maintained their response or remission status for the first 6 months. Subsequently, two patients relapsed, one at 8 months and one at 9 months. The total observation period for individual patients ranged from 7 to 23 months. Although the data from these two studies are further supported by increasing clinical experience using TMS for maintenance purposes after ECT, definitive trials are needed to clarify the value of this approach.

TMS VERSUS ECT: COST-EFFECTIVENESS

Jin et al. (2016) reported that TMS was less costly than ECT ($P<0.05$) and concluded, based on both clinical outcome and economic data, that TMS might be an alternative to ECT for some patients. In contrast, however, a group of researchers from Spain used a probabilistic sensitivity analysis, populating their model with data from various comparison trials of TMS and ECT (Vallejo-Torres et al. 2015). The primary outcome was quality-adjusted life years over a 12-month period. The authors concluded that ECT alone is likely to be a more cost-effective option than TMS alone or TMS followed by ECT, although this last strategy was the most clinically effective.

TMS Versus ECT: Patient Preference

In a retrospective medical record review, Magnezi et al. (2016) considered 81 patients with treatment-resistant major depression who had received TMS or ECT and found a trend in the group effect favoring ECT over TMS. Notably, however, the ECT patients experienced more adverse events, and TMS patients rated their treatment more favorably.

Summary

There has not yet been a definitive, rigorously designed study using the optimal application of TMS for comparison with ECT. Thus, the existing data must be considered preliminary. Nevertheless, there is an increasing clinical utilization of TMS as a substitute or complementary strategy for patients deemed appropriate candidates for ECT, partly driven by patient preference. In the absence of better data, the existing literature indicates that at least a subgroup of depressed patients referred for ECT could potentially benefit from TMS as an alternative, especially if delivered using present-day treatment protocols. More clearly identifying this population is an important next step (Table 7–3).

Clinical Vignette

The patient is a 42-year-old man with a 10-year history of treatment-resistant depression. After multiple failed medication trials and two hospitalizations, he fully recovered after a course of 12 bilateral ECT treatments. Rapid and repeated relapse, however, necessitated the use of maintenance ECT at a frequency of once every 2–3 weeks. Cognitive side effects interfered with the patient's ability to work as a registered nurse for 3–4 days after each treatment. He then underwent a brief series of 10 consecutive daily left-sided 10-Hz TMS treatments, after which he was transitioned to maintenance TMS with one session every 2 weeks for 12 weeks. Treatment frequency was then decreased to once a month, allowing him to remain symptom free and to function at full capacity. After 6 months, sessions were administered on an as-needed basis. He remained in remission and off medication for 24 months with a single TMS treatment every 3 months.

Table 7–3. Comparison of transcranial magnetic stimulation (TMS) and electroconvulsive therapy (ECT)

TMS	ECT
Advantages	
No seizure necessary, no anesthesia, no cognitive disruption	75 years of clinical and research experience
No drug interactions	Often rapidly effective for more severe episodes of depression (e.g., with psychosis, catatonia, high suicidality)
Minimal systemic effects	
Subjects remain independent	
Patient preference	Effective for various disorders (e.g., unipolar and bipolar depression, mania, schizophrenia)
	Minimal systemic effects
Disadvantages	
Limited clinical experience	Access
Time intensive	Patient acceptance/stigma
Relatively slow onset of efficacy	Optimal administration
Application site pain/discomfort	Cost
Potential for seizure	Relapse rates
Cost	Adverse effects (e.g., cognitive)

Other Neuromodulation Treatments for Depression

FOCAL ELECTRICALLY ADMINISTERED SEIZURE THERAPY

FEAST is an experimental form of ECT that uses a unidirectional electrical current along with asymmetrically sized electrodes to more precisely stimulate brain areas involved in depression, including the right orbitofrontal cortex. FEAST produces a focal rather than generalized seizure and thereby causes fewer cognitive side effects than traditional ECT (Sahlem et al. 2016).

MAGNETIC SEIZURE THERAPY

MST may be thought of as a form of TMS intentionally designed to cause a seizure. Because magnetic fields are not affected by scalp/skull resistance, the induced electrical fields are more focal. Preliminary evidence suggests fewer cognitive side effects with MST than with ECT, perhaps because intracerebral current path and density can be better controlled with MST, thus avoiding deeper cortical areas associated with memory (Polster et al. 2015).

A systematic review of eight studies ($N=121$; four controlled comparisons with ECT and four open-label trials) that primarily involved patients with unipolar depression, although a small number of patients with bipolar depression were also included, was undertaken (Cretaz et al. 2015). Although the authors reported substantial benefit with MST (e.g., remission rates ranging from 30% to 40%), the benefits were not as robust as with ECT (e.g., remission rates ranging from 50% to 70%). Notably, however, cognitive adverse effects were far less evident in the MST group. The MST procedure produces a seizure and is painful, and therefore general anesthesia is required. Significant engineering obstacles also need to be overcome because magnetic stimulation is a very inefficient means of inducing a seizure.

VAGUS NERVE STIMULATION

VNS involves the surgical implantation of a matchbox-sized, lithium battery–powered generator under the skin of the patient's chest. This device is attached to the left vagus nerve by a subcutaneous wire with two electrodes. Electrical pulses provide afferent stimulation of the median raphe nucleus, locus coeruleus, and nigrostriatal area, leading to increased serotonergic, adrenergic, and dopaminergic activity. Stimulus settings can be adjusted using an external computerized handheld device. Although VNS has FDA clearance, insurance coverage is rare. Because VNS is a costly and invasive procedure with a delayed onset of effect, it is generally considered a treatment of last resort (Cimpianu et al. 2017).

A few reports exist on the combined use of TMS with implanted vagus nerve stimulators in patients with treatment-resistant depression. One study assessed the risk of inducing currents in the VNS stimulating electrodes with the potential for left vagal nerve damage, heating or movement of VNS components, and unintended change in VNS parameters (Philip et al. 2014). Because the ferromagnetic elements of VNS lie outside the TMS magnetic field, it appears that combining TMS and VNS can be done safely.

Promising preliminary data with transcutaneous auricular vagus nerve stimulation (taVNS) may ultimately help to allay the safety concerns of clinicians noted above and may prompt augmentation studies using the combination of TMS and taVNS (Rong et al. 2016).

DEEP BRAIN STIMULATION

DBS consists of a surgically implanted pulse generator and a wire attached to electrodes that stimulate specific brain nuclei. It has been used primarily for treatment of Parkinson's disease, but there is evidence that it may also be of benefit for other disorders, including treatment-resistant depression. Several targets for DBS treatment of depression are being investigated, but at this time the treatment remains experimental (Narang et al. 2016).

The use of TMS in the presence of an implanted DBS device raises certain safety issues and should be considered a contraindication until further studies can be conducted (see Chapter 3, "Risk Management Issues in Transcranial Magnetic Stimulation for Treatment of Major Depression").

TRANSCRANIAL DIRECT CURRENT STIMULATION

tDCS is a noninvasive technique that applies a small (1–2 mA) direct current via scalp electrodes to enhance or diminish neuronal excitability without causing depolarization. It is safe, inexpensive, easy to administer, and suitable for home use. Preliminary data suggest that it may have some antidepressant effects, but controlled studies report inconsistent findings and any benefit for treatment-resistant depression remains unclear (Brunoni et al. 2013).

CRANIAL ELECTROTHERAPY STIMULATION

Cranial electrotherapy stimulation uses a pulsed electrical current of about 50 µA to 5 mA at a frequency of 100 Hz via surface electrodes on the infra- or supra-auricular areas. It is safe, inexpensive, and suitable for home use. It has had FDA safety clearance since 1978, but controlled studies demonstrating efficacy are lacking. Preliminary data suggest that it may have some antidepressant effects but that any benefit in treatment-resistant depression is likely to be limited (Kavirajan et al. 2014).

EPIDURAL PREFRONTAL CORTICAL STIMULATION

Epidural prefrontal cortical stimulation is an invasive treatment that uses implanted stimulating paddles that target the anterior frontal poles and lateral prefrontal cortex. Preliminary evidence suggests that it is a relatively well-tolerated and possibly effective therapy in some cases of treatment-resistant depression (Williams et al. 2016).

EXTERNAL TRIGEMINAL NERVE STIMULATION

External trigeminal nerve stimulation is a noninvasive treatment in which patch electrodes are placed on the forehead during sleep. Preliminary evidence suggests some antidepressant effect via afferent stimulation of the locus coeruleus (Cook et al. 2013).

Conclusion

Neuromodulation—the therapeutic modification of brain activity using electrical or magnetic energy—can be accomplished by a variety of methods, both invasive and noninvasive. A number of neuromodulation treatments for depression have been developed in recent years. Although many of these treatments remain experimental, electroconvulsive therapy (ECT) and TMS have proven efficacy. Because of the advantages of TMS over ECT, its use has increased significantly.

Evidence suggests that TMS may be as effective as ECT for many patients with nonpsychotic, treatment-resistant major depressive disorder. There is a need for evidence-based guidelines to help clinicians select the treatment that is most likely to be effective. Until studies unveil valid biological markers to better define these populations, clinical markers may provide some guidance. Thus, patients with nonpsychotic, treatment-resistant depression who are not highly suicidal, who are able to meet their basic needs, and who have strong support systems to help monitor their status are candidates for TMS.

KEY CLINICAL POINTS

- TMS is an effective and well-tolerated neuromodulation procedure for treatment-resistant depression.

- TMS may be a preferred alternative to electroconvulsive therapy (ECT) for acute treatment of major depressive disorder in some patients.

- TMS may be used as a complementary treatment to ECT for acute treatment of major depressive disorder.

- TMS may be used as a maintenance treatment after successful completion of an acute course of ECT.

- TMS may play a complementary role with other neuromodulation approaches.

References

Brunoni AR, Valiengo L, Baccaro A, et al: The sertraline vs. electrical current therapy for treating depression clinical study: results from a factorial, randomized, controlled trial. JAMA Psychiatry 70(4):383–391, 2013 23389323

Cimpianu CL, Strube W, Falkai P, et al: Vagus nerve stimulation in psychiatry: a systematic review of the available evidence. J Neural Transm (Vienna) 124(1):145–158, 2017 27848034

Cook IA, Schrader LM, Degiorgio CM, et al: Trigeminal nerve stimulation in major depressive disorder: acute outcomes in an open pilot study. Epilepsy Behav 28(2):221–226, 2013 23773978

Cretaz E, Brunoni AR, Lafer B: Magnetic seizure therapy for unipolar and bipolar depression: a systematic review. Neural Plast 2015:521398, 2015 26075100

Cristancho MA, Helmer A, Connolly R, et al: Transcranial magnetic stimulation maintenance as a substitute for maintenance electroconvulsive therapy: a case series. J ECT 29(2):106–108, 2013 23519219

Dannon PN, Dolberg OT, Schreiber S, et al: Three and six-month outcome following courses of either ECT or rTMS in a population of severely depressed individuals—preliminary report. Biol Psychiatry 51(8):687–690, 2002 11955470

Eranti S, Mogg A, Pluck G, et al: A randomized, controlled trial with 6-month follow-up of repetitive transcranial magnetic stimulation and electroconvulsive therapy for severe depression. Am J Psychiatry 164(1):73–81, 2007 17202547

Grunhaus L, Dannon PN, Schreiber S, et al: Repetitive transcranial magnetic stimulation is as effective as electroconvulsive therapy in the treatment of nondelusional major depressive disorder: an open study. Biol Psychiatry 47(4):314–324, 2000 10686266

Grunhaus L, Schreiber S, Dolberg OT, et al: A randomized controlled comparison of electroconvulsive therapy and repetitive transcranial magnetic stimulation in severe and resistant nonpsychotic major depression. Biol Psychiatry 53(4):324–331, 2003 12586451

Hansen PE, Ravnkilde B, Videbech P, et al: Low-frequency repetitive transcranial magnetic stimulation inferior to electroconvulsive therapy in treating depression. J ECT 27(1):26–32, 2011 20351570

Janicak PG, Dowd SM, Martis B, et al: Repetitive transcranial magnetic stimulation versus electroconvulsive therapy for major depression: preliminary results of a randomized trial. Biol Psychiatry 51(8):659–667, 2002 11955466

Janicak PG, Dowd SM, Strong MJ: The potential role of repetitive transcranial magnetic stimulation in treating severe depression. Psychiatr Ann 35(2):138–145 2005

Jelovac A, Kolshus E, McLoughlin DM: Relapse following successful electroconvulsive therapy for major depression: a meta-analysis. Neuropsychopharmacology 38(12):2467–2474, 2013 23774532

Jin XL, Xu WQ, Le YJ, et al: Long-term effectiveness of modified electroconvulsive therapy compared with repetitive transcranial magnetic stimulation for treatment of recurrent major depressive disorder. J Nerv Ment Dis 204(6):479–482, 2016 26915018

Kavirajan HC, Lueck K, Chuang K: Alternating current cranial electrotherapy stimulation (CES) for depression. Cochrane Database Syst Rev (7):CD010521, 2014 25000907

Kellner CH, Knapp RG, Petrides G, et al: Continuation electroconvulsive therapy vs pharmacotherapy for relapse prevention in major depression: a multisite study from the Consortium for Research in Electroconvulsive Therapy (CORE). Arch Gen Psychiatry 63(12):1337–1344, 2006 17146008

Kellner CH, Husain MM, Knapp RG, et al; CORE/PRIDE Work Group: A novel strategy for continuation ECT in geriatric depression: phase 2 of the PRIDE study. Am J Psychiatry 173(11):1110–1118, 2016 27418381

Keshtkar M, Ghanizadeh A, Firoozabadi A: Repetitive transcranial magnetic stimulation versus electroconvulsive therapy for the treatment of major depressive disorder, a randomized controlled clinical trial. J ECT 27(4):310–314, 2011 22080240

Magnezi R, Aminov E, Shmuel D, et al: Comparison between neurostimulation techniques repetitive transcranial magnetic stimulation vs electroconvulsive therapy for the treatment of resistant depression: patient preference and cost-effectiveness. Patient Prefer Adherence 4(10):1481–1487, 2016 27536079

Martis B, Alam D, Dowd SM, et al: Neurocognitive effects of repetitive transcranial magnetic stimulation in severe major depression. Clin Neurophysiol 114(6):1125–1132, 2003 12804681

Micallef-Trigona B: Comparing the effects of repetitive transcranial magnetic stimulation and electroconvulsive therapy in the treatment of depression: a systematic review and meta-analysis. Depress Res Treat 2014:135049, 2014 25143831

Narang P, Retzlaff A, Brar K, et al: Deep brain stimulation for treatment-refractory depression. South Med J 109(11):700–703, 2016 27812714

Noda Y, Daskalakis ZJ, Ramos C, et al: Repetitive transcranial magnetic stimulation to maintain treatment response to electroconvulsive therapy in depression: a case series. Front Psychiatry 4:73, 2013 23888145

O'Connor M, Brenninkmeyer C, Morgan A, et al: Relative effects of repetitive transcranial magnetic stimulation and electroconvulsive therapy on mood and memory: a neurocognitive risk-benefit analysis. Cogn Behav Neurol 16(2):118–127, 2003 12799598

Philip NS, Carpenter SL, Carpenter LL, et al: Safe use of repetitive transcranial magnetic stimulation in patients with implanted vagus nerve stimulators. Brain Stimul 7(4):608–612, 2014 24794163

Polster JD, Kayser S, Bewernick BH, et al: Effects of electroconvulsive therapy and magnetic seizure therapy on acute memory retrieval. J ECT 31(1):13–19, 2015 24853650

Pridmore S: Substitution of rapid transcranial magnetic stimulation treatments in a course of electroconvulsive therapy. Depress Anxiety 12(3):118–123, 2000 11126185

Pridmore S, Bruno R, Turnier-Shea Y, et al: Comparison of unlimited numbers of rapid transcranial magnetic stimulation (rTMS) and ECT treatment sessions in major depressive episode. Int J Neuropsychopharmacol. 3(2):129–124 2000 11343589

Ren J, Li H, Palaniyappan L, et al: Repetitive transcranial magnetic stimulation versus electroconvulsive therapy for major depression: a systematic review and meta-analysis. Prog Neuropsychopharmacol Biol Psychiatry 51:181–189, 2014 24556538

Rong P, Liu J, Wang L, et al: Effect of transcutaneous auricular vagus nerve stimulation on major depressive disorder: a nonrandomized controlled pilot study. J Affect Disord 195:172–179, 2016 26896810

Rosa MA, Gattaz WF, Pascual-Leone A, et al: Comparison of repetitive transcranial magnetic stimulation and electroconvulsive therapy in unipolar nonpsychotic refractory depression: a randomized, single-blind study. Int J Neuropsychopharmacol 9(6):667–676, 2006 16923322

Sahlem GL, Short EB, Kerns S, et al: Expanded safety and efficacy data for a new method of performing electroconvulsive therapy: focal electrically administered seizure therapy. J ECT 32(3):197–203, 2016 27379790

Schulze-Rauschenbach SC, Harms U, Schlaepfer TE, et al: Distinctive neurocognitive effects of repetitive transcranial magnetic stimulation and electroconvulsive therapy in major depression. Br J Psychiatry 186:410–416, 2005 15863746

Vallejo-Torres L, Castilla I, González N, et al: Cost-effectiveness of electroconvulsive therapy compared to repetitive transcranial magnetic stimulation for treatment-resistant severe depression: a decision model. Psychol Med 45(7):1459–1470, 2015 25354790

Williams NR, Short EB, Hopkins T, et al: Five-year follow-up of bilateral epidural prefrontal cortical stimulation for treatment-resistant depression. Brain Stimul 9(6):897–904, 2016 27443912

Xie J, Chen J, Wei Q: Repetitive transcranial magnetic stimulation versus electroconvulsive therapy for major depression: a meta-analysis of stimulus parameter effects. Neurol Res 35(10):1084–1091, 2013 23889926

8

Transcranial Magnetic Stimulation for the Treatment of Other Mood Disorders

Scott T. Aaronson, M.D.
Paul E. Croarkin, D.O., M.S.

In 2008, the U.S. Food and Drug Administration (FDA) cleared repetitive transcranial magnetic stimulation (TMS) for treatment of major depressive disorder (MDD) in adults failing to receive benefit from antidepressant medications. Additional research and clinical practice confirmed the safety and efficacy of TMS in MDD (George et al. 2010), and clinicians and researchers rapidly began exploring the utility of TMS for other populations. Early work suggests that this noninvasive form of brain stimulation may be beneficial for other indications, such as bipolar depression (Dell'Osso et al. 2011), perinatal depression (Kim et al. 2015), adolescent depression (Donaldson et al. 2014), and late-life depression (Blumberger et al. 2015), thereby offering new options to impaired populations with limited effective therapeutics.

Bipolar depression is pathophysiologically distinct from unipolar depression, carries a substantial disease burden, and has an inadequate evidence base to guide clinical treatment. Furthermore, recent drug development efforts for bipolar depression have concentrated on second-generation antipsychotics, which have an unacceptable side-effect burden for long-term use. *Perinatal depression* is a common and impairing condition that unfortunately is often undertreated. *Depression in adolescence* is a global public health problem contributing to academic failure, delays in social development, substance use, teen pregnancy, and completed suicide. Current treatment options for adolescent depression, which rely primarily on selective serotonin reuptake inhibitors (SSRIs) and evidence-based psychotherapeutic approaches such as cognitive-behavioral therapy (CBT), are often ineffective. *Late-life depression* is frequently undiagnosed; however, even when it is properly identified and treated, it follows a more insidious course than depression in younger populations.

In this chapter, we survey recent research and clinical experience focused on the use of TMS in bipolar depression, perinatal depression, adolescent depression, and late-life depression. Existing information is nascent and larger randomized controlled trials are under way, but initial experience suggests that TMS may be a safe and effective alternative treatment for these indications. Although unique risk factors (e.g., the potential induction of mania and unknown, untoward effects on neurodevelopment) must be carefully considered, the consequences of untreated or inadequately treated depression in bipolar disorder, during the perinatal period, in adolescence, and later in life are significant. Existing knowledge may inform clinicians considering the off-label use of TMS in these populations.

Bipolar Depression

CURRENT TREATMENT PARADIGM

Within the scope of mood disorders, bipolar depression is especially difficult to manage. Treatment practice typically utilizes antidepressants combined with mood-stabilizing agents, despite the absence of clear evidence supporting efficacy of such treatment. Findings from the National Institute of Mental Health–funded Systematic Treatment Enhancement

Program for Bipolar Disorder (STEP-BD), a large study that sought to identify best treatment practices in bipolar disorder, supported the notion that antidepressants added to mood stabilizers do not improve outcomes and may even carry the risk of precipitating a mixed or manic episode (El-Mallakh et al. 2015; Truman et al. 2007).

The International Society for Bipolar Disorder published a consensus statement about the use of antidepressants in bipolar depression (Pacchiarotti et al. 2013), citing the striking incongruity of their wide use despite a weak evidence base for both safety and efficacy. Although the panel did not endorse the use of antidepressants, it did suggest that SSRIs and bupropion may have a lower risk than aminergic agents such as tricyclic antidepressants or serotonin-norepinephrine reuptake inhibitors in causing a manic switch and that patients with bipolar I depression are at higher risk than patients with bipolar II depression for negative outcomes.

The current FDA-approved evidence base for the treatment of bipolar depression is limited to three second-generation antipsychotics, one of which is paired with an SSRI (i.e., quetiapine, lurasidone, and olanzapine plus fluoxetine) (Nierenberg et al. 2015). Their high side-effect burden (especially weight gain, sedation, and metabolic syndrome) makes them an unacceptable choice for many patients. One of the problems in developing safe and effective treatments for bipolar depression is that this population is quite heterogeneous, with subgroups that possibly require different pharmacological interventions (Altshuler et al. 2003; Goldberg et al. 2015).

Another problem with the use of antidepressants is that it is hard, if not impossible, to target only one pole of a cyclical disorder with medications impacting nerve cells and receptor sites over extended periods of time. For patients with rapid-cycling bipolar disorder, continued use of antidepressants was found to be associated with worse outcomes (El-Mallakh et al. 2015). This raises the question as to whether neurostimulation such as TMS can provide briefer, episode-based interventions for bipolar depression without the risk of manic switches or mood destabilization.

EVIDENCE BASE FOR TMS IN BIPOLAR DEPRESSION: RANDOMIZED SHAM-CONTROLLED TRIALS AND A META-ANALYSIS

Although interest in the use of TMS to treat bipolar depression extends back two decades, the development of a clear evidence base is hampered by the lack of cohesiveness in the treatment paradigms used across multiple small studies. Studies have looked at left-sided high-frequency stimulation (>5 Hz), right-sided low-frequency stimulation (1 Hz), and sequential bilateral stimulation over the dorsolateral pre-frontal cortex (DLPFC), with treatment course durations varying between 2 and 4 weeks. A meta-analysis looking at 19 different randomized clinical trials in patients with bipolar disorder (N=181) demonstrated efficacy for right-sided low-frequency stimulation and left-sided high-frequency stimulation but not for sequential bilateral stimulation (McGirr et al. 2016). Another heartening statistic was the very low rate of mood switching, with no significant difference between sham-controlled and active treatment groups (0.9% active vs. 1.3% sham) and no significant adverse events. A more recent study of 49 patients with bipolar and unipolar depression also did not find efficacy for sequential bilateral treatment (Fitzgerald et al. 2016), but this protocol used a very low number of pulses (i.e., 1,000, which is about one-third the normal dose) for each session of left-sided treatment, which may account for a diminished response rate. Another study (N=30) comparing right-sided low-frequency treatment with sequential bilateral treatment found that the latter produced a higher response rate (i.e., 80% vs. 47%) but an equal remission rate (i.e., 40%) (Kazemi et al. 2016).

A randomized sham-controlled trial of deep TMS using the H1 coil in 50 patients with bipolar depression (20 treatments at 18 Hz with 55 two-second trains) showed a statistically significant separation by change in rating scale score (P=0.03), only a trend in categorical rate of response (P=0.08), and no separation by remission at 8-week follow-up (Tavares et al. 2017).

The existing evidence base is heterogeneous for treatment delivery, type of bipolar disorder (e.g., I or II), and use of concomitant medication (subjects were generally not taking antidepressants but may have been taking mood stabilizers, depending on the study). There does, however, appear to be a trend that unilateral treatment (either left-sided high-frequency or right-sided low-frequency) may be more effective than sequential bilateral stimulation for bipolar depression. However, there has not been a head-to-head trial to guide clinicians on the most optimal stimulation protocol, and there is a need for larger trials with better defined homogeneous populations and unified treatment paradigms.

CLINICAL EXPERIENCE WITH TMS IN BIPOLAR DEPRESSION: OPEN-LABEL TRIALS AND CASE REVIEWS

Clinicians providing TMS to patients for bipolar depression have reported varied results, likely due, in part, to population heterogeneity and varying treatment parameters. A summary of the larger cohorts (with more than 10 patients) is provided in Table 8–1.

In a retrospective study of 100 consecutive patients treated for depression in a university-based TMS clinic, Connolly et al. (2012) reported a 35% response rate and a 15% remission rate in the 20 patients with bipolar depression treated for 6 weeks with adjunctive TMS. The treatment was well tolerated, and there were no reports of manic symptoms, but the overall response and remission rates were lower in this subgroup than in the patients with major depression.

In the largest study to date, a retrospective analysis of 39 patients with bipolar I or II depression treated at a specialized hospital-based TMS clinic, Aaronson and Daddario (2016) found higher response rates in the bipolar group than in the unipolar group. All patients were treated with left-sided high-frequency stimulation at 10 Hz, the standard protocol for major depression. Every patient was taking at least one mood stabilizer, and four of the patients with bipolar II disorder continued taking antidepressant medication. All patients had experienced at least two and up to six adequate medication trial failures for their depressive episodes. For the patients with bipolar I disorder, the response rate was 72% (13/18) and the remission rate was 44% (8/18). For the patients with bipolar II disorder, the response rate was 67% (14/21) and the remission rate was 28% (5/18). These data are shown in Figure 8–1.

Agitation leading to discontinuation was seen in 17% (3/18) of the bipolar I group and 5% (1/21) of the bipolar II group. The agitation occurred within the first 2 weeks of treatment and did not meet criteria for mania or hypomania. Among those achieving remission, the average number of treatments to remission was 22. Compared with the 175 patients with unipolar depression treated at the same center, the patients with bipolar disorder had a higher average remission rate (36% vs. 31%), higher response rate (69% vs. 62%), and shorter course to remission (i.e., 22 vs. 29 sessions). Other than agitation there were no significant adverse events.

OPEN QUESTIONS

As often happens in medicine, the clinical use of TMS in bipolar depression has outpaced the creation of a clear evidence base to support the safest and most effective use of this intervention. For a population as clinically underserved as individuals with bipolar depression, TMS may indeed offer a nonpharmacological treatment option that can be used episodically for depressive mood episodes and with a remarkably

Table 8-1. Open-label transcranial magnetic stimulation studies in bipolar depression (N > 10)

Reference	N	Treatment location; coil type	Frequency; intensity; pulses/day	Sessions	Outcomes; measurement	Side effects
Dell'Osso et al. 2009	11	R-DLPFC; Figure eight	1 Hz; 110% MT; 300 pulses	15 over 3 weeks	54.5% response, 36.4% remission; HDRS	No mania/hypomania
Harel et al. 2011	19	L-DLPFC; H coil	20 Hz; 120% MT; 1,680 pulses	20 over 4 weeks	52.6% response, 63.2% remission; HDRS	No mania/hypomania One generalized seizure
Connolly et al. 2012	20	L-DLPFC; Figure eight	10 Hz; 120% MT; 3,000 pulses	30 over 6 weeks	35% response, 15% remission; CGI	No serious adverse events
Aaronson and Daddario 2016	39	L-DLPFC; Figure eight	10 HZ; 120% MT; 3,000 pulses	Up to 30 over 6 weeks	BP1: 44% response, 72% remission BP2: 67% response, 27% remission; MADRS	Treatment-emergent agitation in 17% of BP1 and 5% of BP2 No mania/hypomania

Note. BP1 = patients with bipolar I disorder; BP2 = patients with bipolar II disorder; CGI = Clinical Global Impression Scale; HDRS = Hamilton Depression Rating Scale; L-DLPFC = left dorsolateral prefrontal cortex; MADRS = Montgomery-Åsberg Depression Rating Scale; MT = motor threshold; R-DLPFC = right dorsolateral prefrontal cortex.

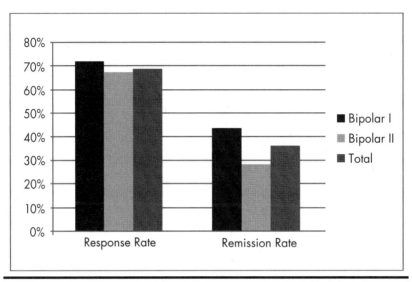

Figure 8–1. Response and remission rates in patients with bipolar I and II depression.

Source. Adapted from Aaronson and Daddario 2016.

benign side-effect profile compared with systemically administered medications. However, some questions remain:

1. What is the optimal stimulation protocol, treatment duration and frequency, and magnetic coil positioning for patients with bipolar depression? Would right-sided low-frequency stimulation be more effective than left-sided high-frequency stimulation? Should different treatment parameters (e.g., length of session, course of treatment, 5- vs. 8- vs. 10-Hz stimulation frequency) be used for bipolar depression than for unipolar depression?
2. Should TMS be administered with medications? Should treatment be given with or without mood stabilizers? Should patients stop taking antidepressants before TMS is initiated? Should patients with bipolar I disorder and those with bipolar II disorder receive different treatments?

TREATMENT CONSIDERATIONS AND RECOMMENDATIONS

Table 8–2 lists treatment considerations and recommendations that have been extrapolated from the existing evidence and clinical experience with the management of bipolar disorder, as well as from TMS treatment of unipolar depression.

Table 8–2. Treatment considerations and recommendations for transcranial magnetic stimulation (TMS) in bipolar depression

Establish a clear diagnosis with regard to the phase of the bipolar illness. Patients with bipolar I disorder are at higher risk for mixed or manic switches than are patients with bipolar II disorder and may need more protection with mood stabilizer support. Generally, patients in the mixed or manic phase of bipolar disorder are not good candidates for TMS, and there is no evidence to support its use. It is also doubtful that TMS can alleviate psychotic symptoms.

Consider mood stabilizer support. History of each patient's illness should help guide clinical decisions. Patients with higher risk of cycling or intensity of mania may do better with lithium or valproate plus a second-generation antipsychotic. Patients with low risk of instability may be managed with lamotrigine. Patients should take a mood stabilizer for a minimum of 2 weeks before starting TMS.

Remember that antidepressants may be problematic. There is no clear evidence to support the use of antidepressants in this population. Give the patient at least 1–2 weeks to taper off antidepressants.

Evaluate patients with bipolar disorder at least weekly while they are receiving TMS. This population is at higher risk for manic switches and is more likely to see earlier response and remission. Furthermore, these patients are at risk for premature discontinuation of TMS secondary to treatment-emergent agitation. Consider using the Young Mania Rating Scale (YMRS) and the Generalized Anxiety Disorder 7-item scale (GAD-7) to monitor for treatment-emergent agitation or subsyndromal manic symptoms. Use a depression rating scale such as the Montgomery-Åsberg Depression Rating Scale (MADRS) to determine severity of illness, and consider stopping TMS if remission criteria are met or if improvement has plateaued for 2 weeks after at least 25 treatments.

Keep in mind that treatment parameters do not have a clear evidence base. The meta-analysis supported benefit for right-sided low-frequency and left-sided high-frequency treatment, but the evidence to justify sequential bilateral treatment was less clear (McGirr et al. 2016). Most TMS centers use the same parameters for bipolar depression as for unipolar depression—that is, left-sided high-frequency stimulation.

Collect data and measure symptom improvement with both patient questionnaires and validated clinician rating scales. The more extensive the clinical experience, the more information can be gathered to optimize treatment with TMS in patients with bipolar depression.

CLINICAL VIGNETTE

The patient is a 40-year-old single woman who is a successful entrepreneur. She has been depressed for the past 6 months and mostly housebound because of her symptoms. Trials of several antidepressants from different classes were unsuccessful because of lack of response at adequate dose and duration or intolerable agitation and insomnia. Her initial diagnosis was unipolar depression, but consultation indicated a long history of psychomotor agitation, decreased need for sleep, and frequent racing thoughts. One parent also had a history of bipolar disorder. Subsequent interviews elicited that the patient has a complex pattern of cycling in her work: she is unable to function for months at a time but then has weeks of extreme productivity, somewhat marred by a pressure of speech, a brusque interpersonal style, the ability to function on 2 hours of sleep, and a sharp increase in alcohol consumption. Her diagnosis is changed to bipolar I disorder, and she begins taking lithium. After 4 weeks with an adequate blood level of the medication, her depression persists and she is recommended for a trial of TMS, which is administered over the left DLPFC at 10 Hz. She experiences a significant improvement in mood after 1 week and full remission after 15 sessions, without manic activation. Acute TMS treatment is then tapered. She has minor recurrences of her depression when she returns to work, but she responds to one TMS session every 2 weeks to successfully maintain remission.

Perinatal Depression

Perinatal (antenatal and postpartum) depression is a common disabling condition that is underdiagnosed and undertreated. Treatment is often suboptimal, with the potential for substantial untoward effects on mothers, fetuses, and developing neonates. For example, depression during the perinatal period is associated with problematic lifestyle choices such as nicotine and alcohol use, substandard self-care, and a considerable risk for suicide. All of these factors may present long-term negative consequences for child development given that exposure to maternal depression can create physiological and psychological stressors for the developing fetus or infant. These adverse effects impact placental epigenetic changes, fetal brain development, language development, and mother-infant bonding. Offspring of depressed mothers have an increased risk for depression, anxiety, and functional impairment (Kim et al. 2015; Stewart and Vigod 2016; Susser et al. 2016).

Treatment of perinatal depression typically involves evidence-based psychotherapeutic approaches such as CBT or interpersonal psychotherapy, pharmacotherapy with SSRIs, or the combination of psychotherapy and antidepressants. Lack of access to screening and psychiatric expertise contributes to undertreatment, but studies also demonstrate that mothers are ambivalent about the use of psychotropic medications during pregnancy or while breastfeeding (Kim et al. 2015; Myczkowski et al. 2012; Stewart and Vigod 2016; Susser et al. 2016). Thus, neuromodulation modalities such as TMS may be important options, with advantages including the lack of systemic effects that could theoretically impact a developing fetus or an infant who is breastfeeding. Furthermore, no concurrent medications are administered with TMS, whereas electroconvulsive therapy (ECT) requires anesthetic agents (Kim et al. 2015; Myczkowski et al. 2012).

The existing published literature that focuses on TMS for perinatal depression is summarized in Table 8–3.

Although evidence from case studies and open-label trials must be interpreted with caution, early results are promising and underscore the necessity of further systematic research. Notably, a variety of low- and high-frequency dosing schedules, coil locations, and relatively brief treatment courses have been undertaken in all trimesters, as well as postpartum. Initial results demonstrate good outcomes in terms of depressive symptom improvement and maternal-fetal health. Early experience indicates that after 24 weeks of pregnancy, women receiving TMS should be positioned on their left side with a wedge cushion under the right lower back for a 30-degree tilt to avoid inferior vena cava compression syndrome, thus mitigating supine hypotension (Kim and Wang 2014; Kim et al. 2015). Researchers examined children (mean age=32.4 months; range 16–64 months) of mothers who had received TMS for depression during pregnancy and a control group of children (mean age=29.04 months; range 14–63 months) whose mothers had a history of untreated depression during pregnancy. In the TMS-treated group, two infants had jaundice and one infant had febrile convulsions. In the untreated group, three infants had jaundice and one infant had low birth weight. Mothers treated with TMS reported a perceived language delay in their children, but there was no actual difference when compared with children of untreated mothers. Results suggested that there were no cognitive or motor delays associated with antenatal TMS treatment for depression. Although these early results are encouraging (Eryılmaz et al. 2015; Kim et al. 2015), further systematic studies are warranted. Notably, we could not find any published reports using the deep TMS H-coil system in this population.

Table 8–4 reviews clinical considerations for the use of TMS in treating perinatal depressions.

Table 8–3. Published experience with transcranial magnetic stimulation (TMS) for perinatal depression

Reference	N	Status of pregnancy	Treatment location	Frequency; intensity	Sessions	Outcomes
Nahas et al. 1999	1	Second trimester	L-DLPFC	5 Hz; 100% MT	14	Rapid improvement in depression and anxiety. Delivered healthy infant at term.
Klirova et al. 2008	2	Second trimester	L-DLPFC	High-frequency; 100% MT	15	Healthy term delivery. Venlafaxine 225 mg/day concurrently.
		Third trimester	R-DLPFC	Low-frequency; 100% MT	15	Infant delivered at 36 weeks; mother had 1 week of "irritability" but healthy otherwise.
Zhang and Hu 2009	3	Early pregnancy	Not reported	Not reported	Not reported	"Significant" improvement in depressive symptoms. Uneventful deliveries with healthy infants.
Garcia et al. 2010	9	Postpartum	L-DLPFC	10 Hz; 120% MT	20	Significant improvement in depressive symptoms by week 2 (HDRS-24). 8 patients reached remission by week 4. At 6 months, 7 patients met criteria for remission without further treatment.

Table 8–3. Published experience with transcranial magnetic stimulation (TMS) for perinatal depression *(continued)*

Reference	N	Status of pregnancy	Treatment location	Frequency; intensity	Sessions	Outcomes
Zhang et al. 2010	1	Second trimester (2 treatment courses)	L-DLPFC;	1 Hz; 90% MT	14	Over 3 treatment courses, the patient demonstrated improvement and no adverse events. She gave birth to a healthy baby.
			L-DLPFC plus R-DLPFC	1 Hz; 90% MT	14	
		Third trimester (1 treatment course)	L-DLPFC plus R-DLPFC	1 Hz; 90% MT	8	
Kim et al. 2011	10	Second or third trimester	R-DLPFC	1 Hz; 100% MT	20	7 women responded (HDRS-17). No adverse maternal or fetal events. 4 patients had a mild headache.
Myczkowski et al. 2012	14	Postpartum	L-DLPFC	5 Hz; 120% MT or sham TMS	20	Active TMS yielded improvement at week 6 (HDRS-17). 2 patients had mild scalp pain. No other side effects.

Table 8–3. Published experience with transcranial magnetic stimulation (TMS) for perinatal depression *(continued)*

Reference	N	Status of pregnancy	Treatment location	Frequency; intensity	Sessions	Outcomes
Burton et al. 2014	1	First, second, and third trimesters (maintenance treatment throughout)	Sequential L-DLPFC plus R-DLPFC	10 Hz; 110% MT to L-DLPFC 1 HZ; 110% MT to R-DLPFC	1 every 2 weeks for 4 years	Maintained remission from depression. No adverse effects. Healthy infant.
Hızlı Sayar et al. 2014	30	First, second, and third trimesters	L-DLPFC	25 Hz; 100% MT	18	Significant decrease in mean HDRS-17 scores after treatment. 1 patient withdrew early. No adverse maternal or fetal events.

Note. HDRS-17 and HDRS-24=Hamilton Depression Rating Scale, 17 items and 24 items, respectively; L-DLPFC=left dorsolateral prefrontal cortex; MT=motor threshold; R-DLPFC=right dorsolateral prefrontal cortex.

Table 8–4. Considerations for transcranial magnetic stimulation (TMS) treatment of perinatal depression

---

Perinatal depression is common, impairing, and treatable.

Suboptimal therapy produces substantial negative effects for mothers, developing fetuses, and infants.

Standard approaches are psychotherapy (e.g., cognitive-behavioral therapy, interpersonal therapy), selective serotonin reuptake inhibitors, or a combination of both.

Wellness strategies (exercise, stress management, bolstering family support, assessing family health) are important aspects of treatment.

When possible, exposure to medications and untreated depressive episodes should be minimized.

Preliminary experience with TMS for both antepartum and postpartum depression is encouraging.

The initial evaluation for TMS should include input from family, obstetrician, primary psychiatrist, and a TMS expert.

The limits of the existing evidence base regarding TMS and the risks of untreated depression should be reviewed with patients and families to assist in an informed decision about treatment.

A variety of TMS dosing strategies have been employed with good results in terms of effectiveness, as well as maternal and fetal health.

Right-sided low-frequency TMS might be the optimal approach.

Relatively brief treatment courses (15–20 sessions) may be effective.

Beyond 24 weeks of pregnancy, a 30-degree left tilt position while the patient is receiving TMS might mitigate supine hypotension.

Clinicians delivering TMS may need to employ creative scheduling practices and resources to serve this population in the context of potential antenatal or child care demands.

CLINICAL VIGNETTE

A 29-year-old woman in week 24 of pregnancy presented with severe symptoms of major depression, including low mood, amotivation, anhedonia, initial insomnia, low self-esteem, decreased appetite, and passive suicidal thoughts. Weekly CBT sessions for the prior 2 months had not improved her symptoms. Her partner and family had concerns about her adherence to antenatal care and health maintenance. Even though she had a history of one prior major depressive episode with a good response to fluoxetine, she was not willing to initiate treatment with antidepressant medication during her pregnancy because of concerns about adverse events. At the obstetrician's recommendation, healthy lifestyle interventions and additional family support were instituted, and the patient consulted a psychiatrist with TMS experience. The psychiatrist reviewed the initial evidence for safety and effectiveness of TMS with the patient, her partner, and the patient's obstetrician. The TMS clinician recommended a 4-week course of daily 1-Hz treatments delivered over the right DLPFC. During each session, to avoid supine hypotension, the patient rested on a cushion under her right lower lumbar region for a 30-degree tilt toward her left side. The patient tolerated treatments with no adverse effects. Serial ratings with the Quick Inventory of Depressive Symptomatology—Self Report (QIDS-SR) as well as the patient's and her partner's reports revealed improvement in depressive symptoms. The patient delivered a full-term, healthy female infant with no complications. At postnatal follow-up, the patient was euthymic and both mother and infant were doing well.

Adolescent Depression

Adolescent MDD is a relatively common, heterogeneous, and undertreated disorder. Worldwide, it presents a significant public health problem and is a primary contributing factor to completed suicide, a leading cause of death in this age group. On an individual level, depressive episodes in adolescents also lead to considerable functional impairment, academic struggles, substance use, social dysfunction, teen pregnancy, lifelong disease burden, and exposure to ineffective treatments (Blazer et al. 1994). Evidence-based psychotherapeutic approaches such as CBT and SSRIs are considered first-line treatment approaches; however, up to 40% of youths may not respond to them. Treatment with CBT and SSRIs may also fail to address relevant neurodevelopmental pathophysiology (March et al. 2007). Furthermore, ongoing controversies regarding the safety and effectiveness of antidepressants for MDD in adolescents accentuate the need for alternative treatment options (Cipriani et al. 2016).

Existing published studies of TMS for adolescent depression are reviewed in Table 8–5.

A systematic review concluded that TMS may be an effective and tolerable intervention for treatment-resistant depression (TRD) in adolescents (Donaldson et al. 2014). Reviewed studies, however, consist only of case reports or unblinded, open-label trials with inadequate sample sizes. In general, dosing strategies parallel clinical practice for adults with depression. For example, various published protocols for treating adolescents offered up to 30 sessions of 10-Hz TMS at 80%–120% of motor threshold applied over the left DLPFC. In the majority of studies, TMS was applied adjunctively with psychotropic medications (Donaldson et al. 2014). One recent effort employed a magnetic resonance imag-

Table 8–5. Published experience with transcranial magnetic stimulation for adolescent depression

Reference	N	Mean age (range)	Treatment location	Frequency; intensity	Pulses/ session; stimulus train; number of trains	Sessions	Duration, weeks	Outcomes
Walter et al. 2001	3	16.7 (16–17)	L-DLPFC	10 Hz; 90%–110% MT	1,600 pulses; 40–80 stimulations; 20–40 trains	10	2	2 participants improved based on HDRS. 1 participant had tension headaches during 2 sessions.
Loo et al. 2006	2	16 (16)	L-DLPFC	10 Hz; 110% MT	2,000 pulses; 50 stimulations; 40 trains	29–36	6–11	Improvement based on BDI and MADRS. No adverse effects. Variable adherence to treatment.
Bloch et al. 2008	9	17.2 (16–18)	L-DLPFC	10 Hz; 80% MT	400 pulses; 20 stimulations; 20 trains	14	3	Lower mean depressive symptom severity assessed with BDI and CDRS at end of treatment weeks 1 and 2. Sustained improvement at 1 month. 5 participants reported mild headaches.

Table 8–5. Published experience with transcranial magnetic stimulation for adolescent depression *(continued)*

Reference	N	Mean age (range)	Treatment location	Frequency; intensity	Pulses/ session; stimulus train; number of trains	Sessions	Duration, weeks	Outcomes
Wall et al. 2011	8	16.5 (14–17)	L-DLPFC	10 Hz; 120% MT	3,000 pulses; 40 stimulations; 75 trains	30	8	Improvement in mean depressive symptom severity based on CDRS-R after 10, 20, and 30 treatments and at 6-month follow-up. 1 participant discontinued at first session due to discomfort. No other adverse effects.
Yang et al. 2014	6	18.7 (15–21)	L-DLPFC	10 Hz; 120% MT	3,000 pulses; 40 stimulations; 75 trains	15	3	4 participants responded with 68% decrease in HDRS. Mild scalp discomfort and headaches reported. 2 participants withdrew (1 before first treatment and 1 after second treatment).

Table 8–5. Published experience with transcranial magnetic stimulation for adolescent depression *(continued)*

Reference	N	Mean age (range)	Treatment location	Frequency; intensity	Pulses/ session; stimulus train; number of trains	Sessions	Duration, weeks	Outcomes
Wall et al. 2016	10	15.9 (13–17)	L-DLPFC	10 Hz; 120% MT	3,000 pulses; 40 stimulations; 75 trains	30	8	Improvement in mean depressive symptom severity with CDRS-R after 10, 20, and 30 treatments and at 6-month follow-up. Scalp discomfort, headaches, dizziness, musculoskeletal discomfort, eye twitching, and nausea reported. 1 participant withdrew during first session due to discomfort.

Note. BDI=Beck Depression Inventory; CDRS=Children's Depression Rating Scale; CDRS-R=Children's Depression Rating Scale—Revised; HDRS=Hamilton Depression Rating Scale; L-DLPFC=left dorsolateral prefrontal cortex; MADRS=Montgomery-Åsberg Depression Rating Scale; MT=motor threshold.

ing (MRI)–guided approach for TMS coil localization; however, the added clinical benefit of this approach is uncertain (Wall et al. 2016).

Although these results are encouraging for the application of TMS in adolescent TRD, many unanswered questions and challenges remain. Ideally, future studies and clinical registry efforts will standardize approaches for comparison across sites. A federally funded study of adolescent TRD enrolled patients who failed to respond to 8 weeks of treatment with an SSRI at an adequate dose (40 mg/day of fluoxetine or its equivalent) (McMakin et al. 2012). Consensus on the definition of adolescent TRD is lacking, however, and international guidelines suggest that therapeutic TMS should only be applied in youths for a convincing clinical objective (Rossi et al. 2009). Some adolescents and families might favor the use of TMS over medication, but data to guide this approach are limited. Fortunately, randomized, double-blind, sham-controlled trials are planned or are underway to address existing knowledge gaps. For example, one ongoing study is enrolling patients ages 12–21 years who did not respond to at least one adequate trial of an antidepressant during an episode of MDD (Neuronetics 2017). The study design involves an acute 6-week course comparing active and sham TMS sessions. Participants who do not receive initial clinical benefit will have the opportunity to continue in open-label treatment with active TMS. Participants who benefit will have long-term monitoring with reintroduction of TMS as needed.

Published data on ECT in adolescents suggest that it is a safe and effective treatment for severe, treatment-resistant psychiatric disorders (Puffer et al. 2016). Considerations for referring an adolescent for ECT include the presence of severe depression, bipolar disorder, or schizophrenia spectrum illnesses. In any of these disorders, symptoms should be persistent, severe, and life-threatening. Examples include failure to eat and take fluids, imminent suicidality, catatonia, and psychosis. Symptoms should also demonstrate resistance to at least two optimal trials of appropriate pharmacotherapy with evidence-based psychotherapeutic approaches. In most circumstances, adolescents receiving ECT are hospitalized. Notably, a variety of state and institutional guidelines restrict access to ECT for adolescents in some settings (Ghaziuddin et al. 2004).

More study and experience with ECT and TMS for adolescent depression are needed. In the meantime, clinical factors, pragmatic considerations, and existing literature suggest that these two modalities are treatment options for distinct populations in terms of symptom severity and acuity (Puffer et al. 2016).

With any off-label or investigational therapy, adolescents, families, and clinicians should temper enthusiasm with a careful consideration of the risk-benefit ratio and the limits of existing evidence. Recent commentaries focus on the promise and perils of brain stimulation approaches such as TMS during brain development (Davis 2014; Geddes 2015). The potential differences in myelination, neuroanatomy, and electrical field distributions in youths compared with adults present challenges in anticipating the broad effects of stimulation. Although initial systematic reviews suggest that TMS has a favorable side-effect profile in youths, longer-term data are lacking. Risk of seizure may also be greater in youths than adults, and there are open questions regarding the relative pain and sensitivity to TMS in youths compared with adults. At present, it is also unknown if youths undergoing TMS have an increased risk for suicidal behaviors or mania (Rossi et al. 2009). Furthermore, dosing guidelines are not available to help clinicians in treating adolescents (Davis 2014). A recent case report of an induced seizure with deep TMS also demonstrates the need for future dose-finding research in adolescent depression (Cullen et al. 2016) (see Chapter 3, "Risk Management Issues in Transcranial Magnetic Stimulation for Treatment of Major Depression"). Although neurodevelopmentally informed and translational studies are lacking at present, TMS will likely offer an important treatment option for adolescent depression in the future. It is important, however, to consider that current, ubiquitous, off-label practices with polypharmacy are also poorly understood (Kearns and Hawley 2014) and, compared with TMS, could present a greater side-effect burden and risk for adolescents. Table 8–6 reviews key considerations for clinicians, patients, and families contemplating the use of TMS for depression in adolescents.

CLINICAL VIGNETTE

An 18-year-old woman with a history of recurrent MDD and generalized anxiety disorder dating back to age 11 years presented for treatment. Numerous trials of psychotherapy and adequate trials of psychotropic medications (e.g., fluoxetine, escitalopram, venlafaxine, desvenlafaxine, buspirone, lamotrigine, quetiapine, aripiprazole) guided by prior pharmacogenomic testing were ineffective or poorly tolerated. At the time of consultation, she was taking sertraline 100 mg/day and reported some relief in terms of her anxiety, but she was not comfortable increasing the dose because of side-effect concerns and continued to experience symptoms of depression. Despite a good academic record, she was unable to work or attend college. Her history revealed that at age 14 she had participated in an open-label trial of 10-Hz TMS applied over the left DLPFC. The patient and her parents noted that TMS provided more relief from depressive and anxiety symptoms than any prior medication trials. The treatment team completed the evaluation and successfully advocated for insurance coverage of TMS given her prior response to treatment. The patient continued to take sertraline 100 mg/day and completed a 6-week course of 10-Hz TMS. She had a good clinical response and soon returned to college and part-time work. At follow-up 2 years later, she had maintained her improvement.

Late-Life Depression

Clinical experience indicates that depression is common in elderly adults and that this population is particularly susceptible to treatment resistance, relapse, and recurrence (Blumberger et al. 2015). Owing to the heightened sensitivity to adverse medication effects and drug interactions in this age group, alternative therapies are sorely needed (Gálvez et al. 2015). Although ECT plays an important role in managing late-life depression (LLD), the high relapse rates and deleterious effects on cognition are important critical considerations (Kellner et al. 2016). In efforts to partially fill this therapeutic void while avoiding the complications of existing options, other neuromodulation approaches such as TMS are being considered (see Chapter 3).

Initially, TMS was thought to be less effective for treating LLD, in part because of the increased coil-to-cortex distance due to age-related brain atrophic changes. For example, one study using right-sided, low-frequency, low-pulse TMS reported an inverse relationship between the reduction in baseline Hamilton Depression Rating Scale (HDRS) scores and older age (>60 years) (Pallanti et al. 2012). Another study compared two active TMS groups (i.e., total cumulative dose was either 12,000 or 18,000 pulses) versus a sham control group. Participants were 92 unmedicated patients with MRI-defined vascular depression (Jorge et al. 2008). The authors concluded that frontal atrophy and older age were associated with decreased response to TMS. Such reports, coupled with the exclusion of older patients from many clinical trials, leave unanswered the important question of what role TMS might play in treating LLD.

Regardless, other preliminary evidence is promising and provides some guidance for clinicians considering TMS for their elderly depressed patients. For example, a meta-analysis of TMS for treatment of major depression did not find age to be a mitigating factor in diminishing the efficacy of TMS, in part due to the higher number of pulses and more intense stimulation levels in recent trials (Berlim et al. 2014). In addition, high degrees of safety and tolerability were observed in studies that included older patients (e.g., Janicak et al. 2008). One supportive

Table 8–6. Considerations for transcranial magnetic stimulation (TMS) treatment of adolescent depression

Presently, TMS is used off-label for adolescent depression.

Psychotropic medications are also often prescribed off-label for children and adolescents.

Initial experience suggests that TMS may have a low side-effect burden in adolescents.

Long-term safety studies of TMS in adolescents are lacking.

Baseline and follow-up assessment of symptom severity should include standardized rating scales.

A comprehensive treatment history should be obtained to evaluate prior interventions and adherence.

Comorbidity should be assessed and carefully considered.

Historical suicidal behavior should be characterized, and current suicidality should be evaluated.

Patients with *mild symptom severity* often respond to psychoeducation, supportive interventions, and adequate trials of evidence-based psychotherapies such as CBT or IPT.

Patients with *moderate to severe symptom severity* often respond to pharmacotherapy, evidence-based psychotherapies such as CBT and IPT, or their combination.

At a minimum, treatment resistance should be defined in the context of an adequate prior antidepressant trial (e.g., fluoxetine 20–40 mg/day for at least 8 weeks).

Suicidality should be assessed carefully during any treatment.

A meticulous informed consent process for adolescents and parents is imperative. This should impart understanding of the relevant limits of the evidence base for TMS in adolescents and the paucity of long-term safety data. Off-label practices with antidepressant medications and polypharmacy can be discussed in this context to compare evidence bases and potential tolerability.

Patient and parent preferences should be carefully considered.

Extant published experience in adolescent depression primarily involves 10-Hz TMS applied over the left dorsolateral prefrontal cortex.

Prior studies of TMS in adolescent depression often applied TMS as an "adjunctive" treatment to pharmacotherapy in small samples of participants.

Table 8–6. Considerations for transcranial magnetic stimulation (TMS) treatment of adolescent depression *(continued)*

Landmark studies of adults with depression have applied TMS as a monotherapy.

Interindividual variation in motor threshold intensity is common, but younger teenagers often have higher motor threshold intensities.

Initial titration of treatment intensity (e.g., from 80% to 120% over 4–5 days) may improve tolerability for adolescents.

Note. CBT=cognitive-behavioral therapy; IPT=interpersonal therapy.

example is a recent 4-week, double-blind, sham-controlled study from China that included 178 medicated depressed elderly patients (Qin et al. 2017). Although symptoms improved for patients in both treatment arms, the active TMS group, compared with the sham TMS group, experienced a faster onset in overall benefit and greater reduction in suicidal ideation ($P<0.01$) in the first 2 weeks and a higher response rate (i.e., 78% vs. 53%; $P<0.5$) after 4 weeks.

Given the pressing need to provide alternative treatment options and the lack of adequate research with TMS for LLD, this is an area in which well-conceived and well-executed trials can produce much clinical value. For now, when treatment of LLD with TMS is being considered, the dose-response relationship appears to be critical in achieving optimal outcomes.

Conclusion

The efficacy of TMS for major depression in adults is clearly established. Further systematic, prospective work will continue to provide clinicians with evidence-based approaches for reintroduction of TMS, novel stimulus dosing methods, and concurrent treatment with other modalities such as psychotherapeutic approaches.

Further research into treatments is needed for populations with bipolar depression, perinatal depression, adolescent depression, and late-life depression because there are limitations in existing treatment modalities for these disorders. Preliminary evidence highlights the potential clinical benefit and safety profile of TMS for these patients, but data from large randomized controlled trials are needed to better inform practice. Many open questions remain regarding the long-term benefit, safety, tolerability, and optimal dosing strategies for patients in these populations. However, given the risks involved in undertreating these disorders, TMS clinicians, treatment teams, families, and patients may opt to pursue thoughtful off-label use of TMS. In these cases, this approach should be guided by existing data and a careful review of the relative unknowns; acknowledgment of the limits in the evidence base; and consideration of the risk-benefit ratios of TMS versus alternative, potentially suboptimal treatments.

KEY CLINICAL POINTS

For bipolar depression

- Bipolar depression has few evidence-based treatments that demonstrate good tolerability.

- Early experience supports the need for further development of an evidence base for the use of TMS in bipolar depression.

- Patients who are taking adequate mood stabilizers and have a persistent depressive episode may be candidates for TMS.

- In the absence of clear treatment guidelines, patients with bipolar depression should be taking at least one mood-stabilizing agent and avoiding antidepressants before TMS therapy is initiated.

- Patients with bipolar depression receiving TMS should be evaluated at least weekly to ascertain efficacy and a possible switch to mania or treatment-emergent agitation.

For perinatal depression

- Perinatal depression is a common disabling condition.

- Suboptimal treatment contributes to untoward effects on mothers, fetuses, and developing neonates.

- Prior research suggests that many patients are not comfortable using antidepressant medications during pregnancy or while breastfeeding.

- Initial experience suggests that TMS may be a safe and effective treatment modality with a favorable side-effect profile.

- Although prior published experience describes both low- and high-frequency TMS dosing for perinatal depression, low-frequency TMS may be a more favorable approach in terms of tolerability and safety.

- At and beyond 24 weeks of pregnancy, a 30-degree pelvic tilt is recommended to avoid supine hypotension.

For adolescent depression

- Currently, TMS has U.S. Food and Drug Administration clearance for adults (ages 22–68) with depression who have not benefited from antidepressant medications. Initial research and limited clinical experience suggest that TMS is also a promising treatment for adolescent depression.

- Existing trials for adolescent depression are open-label and typically involve 10-Hz TMS applied over the left dorsolateral prefrontal cortex with adjunctive psychotropic medications and psychotherapy.

- Although existing evidence suggests that TMS is safe and tolerable for adolescent depression, further neurodevelopmentally informed research is important.

- Clinicians should consider a referral for TMS for an adolescent patient with an episode of major depressive disorder that is inadequately responsive to appropriate trials of selective serotonin reuptake inhibitors and evidence-based psychotherapy such as cognitive-behavioral therapy.

- Families, patients, and clinicians must carefully consider the limits of knowledge and the risk-benefit ratio of TMS.

For late-life depression

- Late-life depression (LLD) is difficult to diagnose.

- Even when depression is properly recognized, elderly patients are often resistant to standard medication treatments and frequently more susceptible to their adverse effects compared with younger individuals.

- Although electroconvulsive therapy (ECT) is an effective acute treatment for LLD, adverse cognitive effects and high relapse rates presently limit its overall effectiveness.

- Neuromodulation approaches such as TMS are being increasingly considered as alternatives to ECT in the clinical arena.

- Presently, there are inadequate research data to confirm a definitive role for TMS in the management of LLD.

- The presence in older adults of atrophic changes in the area of TMS delivery may suggest a lower response rate.

- Although clinicians should be mindful of limitations, the present database indicates that TMS is safe, well tolerated, and possibly efficacious for LLD when the more recent increased-dosing strategies applied in younger patients are used.

References

Aaronson ST, Daddario K: A retrospective analysis of bipolar depression treated with transcranial magnetic stimulation. Presented at the Society of Biological Psychiatry, Atlanta, GA, May 12–14, 2016

Altshuler L, Suppes T, Black D, et al: Impact of antidepressant discontinuation after acute bipolar depression remission on rates of depressive relapse at 1-year follow-up. Am J Psychiatry 160(7):1252–1262, 2003 12832239

Berlim MT, van den Eynde F, Tovar-Perdomo S, et al: Response, remission and drop-out rates following high-frequency repetitive transcranial magnetic stimulation (rTMS) for treating major depression: a systematic review and meta-analysis of randomized, double-blind and sham-controlled trials. Psychol Med 44(2):225–239, 2014 23507264

Blazer DG, Kessler RC, McGonagle KA, et al: The prevalence and distribution of major depression in a national community sample: the National Comorbidity Survey. Am J Psychiatry 151(7):979–986, 1994 8010383

Bloch Y, Grisaru N, Harel EV, et al: Repetitive transcranial magnetic stimulation in the treatment of depression in adolescents: an open-label study. J ECT 24(2):156–159, 2008 18580562

Blumberger DM, Hsu JH, Daskalakis ZJ: A review of brain stimulation treatments for late-life depression. Curr Treat Options Psychiatry 2(4):413–421, 2015 27398288

Burton C, Gill S, Clarke P, et al: Maintaining remission of depression with repetitive transcranial magnetic stimulation during pregnancy: a case report. Arch Womens Ment Health 17(3):247–250, 2014 24638141

Cipriani A, Zhou X, Del Giovane C, et al: Comparative efficacy and tolerability of antidepressants for major depressive disorder in children and adolescents: a network meta-analysis. Lancet 388(10047):881–890, 2016 27289172

Connolly KR, Helmer A, Cristancho MA, et al: Effectiveness of transcranial magnetic stimulation in clinical practice post-FDA approval in the United States: results observed with the first 100 consecutive cases of depression at an academic medical center. J Clin Psychiatry 73(4):e567–e573, 2012 22579164

Cullen KR, Jasberg S, Nelson B, et al: Seizure induced by deep transcranial magnetic stimulation in an adolescent with depression. J Child Adolesc Psychopharmacol 26(7):637–641, 2016 27447245

Davis NJ: Transcranial stimulation of the developing brain: a plea for extreme caution. Front Hum Neurosci 8:600, 2014 25140146

Dell'Osso B, Mundo E, D'Urso N, et al: Augmentative repetitive navigated transcranial magnetic stimulation (rTMS) in drug-resistant bipolar depression. Bipolar Disord 11(1):76–81, 2009 19133969

Dell'Osso B, D'Urso N, Castellano F, et al: Long-term efficacy after acute augmentative repetitive transcranial magnetic stimulation in bipolar depression: a 1-year follow-up study. J ECT 27(2):141–144, 2011 20966770

Donaldson AE, Gordon MS, Melvin GA, et al: Addressing the needs of adolescents with treatment resistant depressive disorders: a systematic review of rTMS. Brain Stimul 7(1):7–12, 2014 24527502

El-Mallakh RS, Vöhringer PA, Ostacher MM, et al: Antidepressants worsen rapid-cycling course in bipolar depression: a STEP-BD randomized clinical trial. J Affect Disord 184:318–321, 2015 26142612

Eryılmaz G, Sayar GH, Özten E, et al: Follow-up study of children whose mothers were treated with transcranial magnetic stimulation during pregnancy: preliminary results. Neuromodulation 18(4):255–260, 2015 25257229

Fitzgerald PB, Hoy KE, Elliot D, et al: A negative double-blind controlled trial of sequential bilateral rTMS in the treatment of bipolar depression. J Affect Disord 198:158–162, 2016 27016659

Gálvez V, Ho KA, Alonzo A, et al: Neuromodulation therapies for geriatric depression. Curr Psychiatry Rep 17(7):59, 2015 25995098

Garcia KS, Flynn P, Pierce KJ, et al: Repetitive transcranial magnetic stimulation treats postpartum depression. Brain Stimul 3(1):36–41, 2010 20633429

Geddes L: Brain stimulation in children spurs hope—and concern. Nature 525(7570):436–437, 2015 26399806

George MS, Lisanby SH, Avery D, et al: Daily left prefrontal transcranial magnetic stimulation therapy for major depressive disorder: a sham-controlled randomized trial. Arch Gen Psychiatry 67(5):507–516, 2010 20439832

Ghaziuddin N, Kutcher SP, Knapp P, et al; Work Group on Quality Issues; AACAP: Practice parameter for use of electroconvulsive therapy with adolescents. J Am Acad Child Adolesc Psychiatry 43(12):1521–1539, 2004 15564821

Goldberg JF, Freeman MP, Balon R, et al: The American Society of Clinical Psychopharmacology survey of psychopharmacologists' practice patterns for the treatment of mood disorders. Depress Anxiety 32(8):605–613, 2015 26129956

Harel EV, Zangen A, Roth Y, et al: H-coil repetitive transcranial magnetic stimulation for the treatment of bipolar depression: an add-on, safety and feasibility study. World J Biol Psychiatry 12(2):119–126, 2011 20854181

Hızlı Sayar G, Ozten E, Tufan E, et al: Transcranial magnetic stimulation during pregnancy. Arch Womens Ment Health 17(4):311–315, 2014 24248413

Janicak PG, O'Reardon JP, Sampson SM, et al: Transcranial magnetic stimulation in the treatment of major depressive disorder: a comprehensive summary of safety experience from acute exposure, extended exposure, and during reintroduction treatment. J Clin Psychiatry 69(2):222–232, 2008 18232722

Jorge RE, Moser DJ, Acion L, et al: Treatment of vascular depression using repetitive transcranial magnetic stimulation. Arch Gen Psychiatry 65(3):268–276, 2008 18316673

Kazemi R, Rostami R, Khomami S, et al: Electrophysiological correlates of bilateral and unilateral repetitive transcranial magnetic stimulation in patients with bipolar depression. Psychiatry Res 240:364–375, 2016 27138833

Kearns MA, Hawley KM: Predictors of polypharmacy and off-label prescribing of psychotropic medications: a national survey of child and adolescent psychiatrists. J Psychiatr Pract 20(6):438–447, 2014 25406048

Kellner CH, Husain MM, Knapp RG, et al; CORE/PRIDE Work Group: A novel strategy for continuation ECT in geriatric depression: phase 2 of the PRIDE study. Am J Psychiatry 173(11):1110–1118, 2016 27418381

Kim DR, Wang E: Prevention of supine hypotensive syndrome in pregnant women treated with transcranial magnetic stimulation. Psychiatry Res 218(1–2):247–248, 2014 24768354

Kim DR, Epperson N, Paré E, et al: An open label pilot study of transcranial magnetic stimulation for pregnant women with major depressive disorder. J Womens Health (Larchmt) 20(2):255–261, 2011 21314450

Kim DR, Snell JL, Ewing GC, et al: Neuromodulation and antenatal depression: a review. Neuropsychiatr Dis Treat 11:975–982, 2015 25897234

Klirova M, Novak T, Kopecek M, et al: Repetitive transcranial magnetic stimulation (rTMS) in major depressive episode during pregnancy. Neuro Endocrinol Lett 29(1):69–70, 2008 18283246

Loo C, McFarquhar T, Walter G: Transcranial magnetic stimulation in adolescent depression. Australas Psychiatry 14(1):81–85, 2006 16630205

March JS, Silva S, Petrycki S, et al: The Treatment for Adolescents with Depression Study (TADS): long-term effectiveness and safety outcomes. Arch Gen Psychiatry 64(10):1132–1143, 2007 17909125

McGirr A, Karmani S, Arsappa R, et al: Clinical efficacy and safety of repetitive transcranial magnetic stimulation in acute bipolar depression. World Psychiatry 15(1):85–86, 2016 26833619

McMakin DL, Olino TM, Porta G, et al: Anhedonia predicts poorer recovery among youth with selective serotonin reuptake inhibitor treatment-resistant depression. J Am Acad Child Adolesc Psychiatry 51(4):404–411, 2012 22449646

Myczkowski ML, Dias AM, Luvisotto T, et al: Effects of repetitive transcranial magnetic stimulation on clinical, social, and cognitive performance in postpartum depression. Neuropsychiatr Dis Treat 8:491–500, 2012 23118543

Nahas Z, Bohning DE, Molloy MA, et al: Safety and feasibility of repetitive transcranial magnetic stimulation in the treatment of anxious depression in pregnancy: a case report. J Clin Psychiatry 60(1):50–52, 1999 10074879

Neuronetics: Safety and effectiveness of NeuroStar® transcranial magnetic stimulation (TMS) therapy in depressed adolescents. ClinicalTrials.gov, February 16, 2017. Available at: https://clinicaltrials.gov/ct2/show/NCT02586688. Accessed April 7, 2017.

Nierenberg AA, McIntyre RS, Sachs GS: Improving outcomes in patients with bipolar depression: a comprehensive review. J Clin Psychiatry 76(3):e10, 2015 25830453

Pacchiarotti I, Bond DJ, Baldessarini RJ, et al: The International Society for Bipolar Disorders (ISBD) task force report on antidepressant use in bipolar disorders. Am J Psychiatry 170(11):1249–1262, 2013 24030475

Pallanti S, Cantisani A, Grassi G, et al: rTMS age-dependent response in treatment-resistant depressed subjects: a mini-review. CNS Spectr 17(1):24–30, 2012 22790115

Puffer CC, Wall CA, Huxsahl JE, et al: A 20 year practice review of electroconvulsive therapy for adolescents. J Child Adolesc Psychopharmacol 26(7):632–636, 2016 26784386

Qin BY, Dai LL, Zheng Y: Efficacy of repetitive transcranial magnetic stimulation for alleviating clinical symptoms and suicidal ideation in elderly depressive patients: a randomized controlled trial [in Chinese]. Nan Fang Yi Ke Da Xue Xue Bao 37(1):97–101, 2017 28109107

Rossi S, Hallett M, Rossini PM, et al; Safety of TMS Consensus Group: Safety, ethical considerations, and application guidelines for the use of transcranial magnetic stimulation in clinical practice and research. Clin Neurophysiol 120(12):2008–2039, 2009 19833552

Stewart DE, Vigod S: Postpartum depression. N Engl J Med 375(22):2177–2186, 2016 27959754

Susser LC, Sansone SA, Hermann AD: Selective serotonin reuptake inhibitors for depression in pregnancy. Am J Obstet Gynecol 215(6):722–730, 2016 27430585

Tavares DF, Myczkowski ML, Alberto RL, et al: Treatment of bipolar depression with deep TMS (dTMS): results from a double-blind, randomized, parallel group, sham-controlled clinical trial. Neuropsychopharmacology Feb 1, 2017 doi: 10.1038/npp.2017.26 28145409

Truman CJ, Goldberg JF, Ghaemi SN, et al: Self-reported history of manic/hypomanic switch associated with antidepressant use: data from the Systematic Treatment Enhancement Program for Bipolar Disorder (STEP-BD). J Clin Psychiatry 68(10):1472–1479, 2007 17960960

Wall CA, Croarkin PE, Sim LA, et al: Adjunctive use of repetitive transcranial magnetic stimulation in depressed adolescents: a prospective, open pilot study. J Clin Psychiatry 72(9):1263–1269, 2011 21951987

Wall CA, Croarkin PE, Maroney-Smith MJ, et al: Magnetic resonance imaging-guided, open-label, high-frequency repetitive transcranial magnetic stimulation for adolescents with major depressive disorder. J Child Adolesc Psychopharmacol 26(7):582–589, 2016 26849202

Walter G, Tormos JM, Israel JA, Pascual-Leone A: Transcranial magnetic stimulation in young persons: a review of known cases. J Child Adolesc Psychopharmacol 11(1):69–75, 2001 11322748

Yang XR, Kirton A, Wilkes TC, et al: Glutamate alterations associated with transcranial magnetic stimulation in youth depression: a case series. J ECT 30(3):242–247, 2014 24820947

Zhang D, Hu Z: rTMS may be a good choice for pregnant women with depression. Arch Womens Ment Health 12(3):189–190, 2009 19238519

Zhang X, Liu K, Sun J, et al: Safety and feasibility of repetitive transcranial stimulation (rTMS) as a treatment for major depressive disorder during pregnancy. Arch Womens Ment Health 13(4):369–370, 2010 20386939

Transcranial Magnetic Stimulation for Disorders Other Than Depression

Jaspreet Pannu, B.Sc.
Danielle D. DeSouza, Ph.D.
Zoe Samara, Ph.D.
Kristin S. Raj, M.D.
Nolan R. Williams, M.D.
Karl I. Lanocha, M.D.

Transcranial magnetic stimulation (TMS) is still experimental when it comes to treating disorders other than depression, but its success for depression has led many to wonder whether it might also be effective for other conditions. After all, "treatment resistance" is common not only in depression but also in schizophrenia, obsessive-compulsive disorder (OCD), posttraumatic stress disorder (PTSD), chronic pain, and many other illnesses. Current pharmacological approaches for these conditions have limitations, and electroconvulsive therapy may produce significant side effects for some patients.

Developing stimulation-based treatments for any disorder begins with delineating the underlying neural circuitry of the disorder. Only with this understanding can researchers identify the key brain regions to target that are 1) involved in the pathophysiology of the disorder and 2) accessible to the depth of stimulation being used. Foundational knowledge of the relevant circuit(s) is also important for hypothesizing how other distinct—and sometimes distant—brain regions may be affected by stimulation.

In this chapter, we discuss how TMS-based treatments show promise for application to complex psychiatric illnesses.

Schizophrenia

AUDITORY VERBAL HALLUCINATIONS

Auditory verbal hallucinations are a hallmark positive symptom of schizophrenia. Imaging studies link hyperactivity of left-sided auditory and linguistic areas of the brain, including the left temporoparietal cortex, left superior temporal cortex, and Broca's area, to the pathophysiology of such hallucinations, providing a potential target for TMS (Silbersweig et al. 1995; see Figure 9–1).

The first report of TMS treatment of auditory hallucinations involved three patients with schizophrenia (Hoffman et al. 1999). Slow-frequency 1-Hz stimulation over the left temporoparietal junction (midway between T3 and P3 electroencephalogram electrode sites) was performed for a maximum of 16 minutes, leading to a decrease in the frequency and intensity of hallucinations. A larger, controlled study lasting 9 days again showed substantial improvement following 1-Hz stimulation over the left temporoparietal cortex. More than half of the patients who improved showed sustained benefit 15 weeks later (Hoffman et al. 2003).

Over 30 studies involving more than 700 patients have since been completed. So far, only 1-Hz stimulation of the left temporoparietal cortex has consistently demonstrated efficacy (Slotema et al. 2014). It is worth noting that some patients improve with short courses of treatment and that improvement may often be sustained by periodic retreatment when symptoms emerge (Fitzgerald et al. 2006).

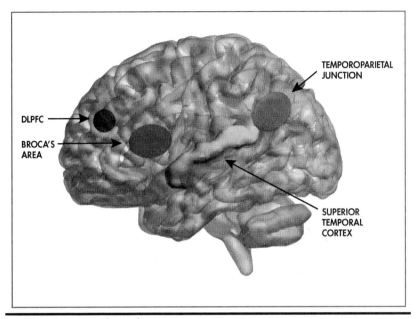

Figure 9–1. Schizophrenia circuit.

See Plate 1 to view this figure in color.

Left-sided lateral view of the brain outlining regions of interest in schizophrenia. The auditory and linguistic areas of the brain responsible for speech, including the right and left superior temporal cortex, Broca's area, and the left temporoparietal area, are implicated in auditory hallucinations. The negative symptoms of schizophrenia are associated with hypoactivity of the dorsolateral prefrontal cortex (DLPFC). Image was visualized with the BrainNet Viewer (Xia et al. 2013).

NEGATIVE SYMPTOMS

Antipsychotic agents of all generations are less effective in reducing negative symptoms, such as flat affect, alogia, anhedonia, and avolition, than positive symptoms. Similar to what is seen in depression, these negative symptoms are associated with hypoactivity of the dorsolateral prefrontal cortex (DLPFC), suggesting that high-frequency stimulation may be of benefit (Stanford et al. 2011). Although a number of studies have used this approach and many of them have found evidence of improvement, they are limited by small sample sizes and short durations of treatment. Another potential confounding variable is that improvement in depression may be misinterpreted as improvement in negative symptoms.

Cole et al. (2015) assessed 10 studies ($N=257$) in which high-frequency TMS targeted the left DLPFC with the aim of increasing cortical excitation and inducing dopamine release. Effect sizes ranged from 0.58 to 0.63

when all trials (including open-label trials) were included. Because effect sizes for antipsychotic medication treatment of negative symptoms range from 0.17 to 0.21, TMS may be an appropriate treatment for some patients (Slotema et al. 2010).

CLINICAL VIGNETTE

The patient is a 24-year-old single woman with schizophrenia. She was living at home with her parents and being treated at a clinic specializing in treatment of early-onset psychosis. Symptoms developed during her first year of college, when she began hearing voices and believed that her thoughts were controlled by robots. She was hospitalized and unable to continue her education. She abandoned her interests and withdrew from family and friends. Her thinking was disorganized and her concentration poor. She could not sit through a movie and had not driven for several years. In public settings, she displayed poor impulse control and was often inappropriate, intrusive, and prone to arguments with strangers.

At the time of evaluation, she was taking lurasidone 60 mg/day. Previous treatments included risperidone, olanzapine, and aripiprazole, which were of limited benefit and poorly tolerated because of weight gain and sedation. Her Positive and Negative Syndrome Scale (PANSS) score was 91 and her Quick Inventory of Depressive Symptomatology—Self-Report (QIDS-SR) score was 7. She denied auditory hallucinations, and there was no clear evidence of delusions, but she was highly distractible, restless, and unable to sit still for more than a few minutes.

She underwent a course of 26 left-sided high-frequency treatments at 10 Hz. During the first week of treatment, she was restless, was easily distracted, and could not remain in the treatment chair for more than about 10 minutes at a time. By the end of her second week, she was able to sit through an entire treatment without interruption. During week 4, she drove herself to treatment with one of her parents in the car. At the end of treatment, her restlessness had completely subsided, her focusing ability had significantly improved, and she had resumed her interest in music and dance. She took responsibility for scheduling her own appointments and was planning to resume college on a part-time basis. Her PANSS and QIDS-SR scores were 56 and 3, respectively. Improvement was sustained when she was seen in follow-up 12 weeks later.

Obsessive-Compulsive Disorder

Up to 60% of patients with OCD experience persistent symptoms despite medications and psychotherapy (Pallanti and Quercioli 2006). Evidence suggests that the orbitofronto-striato-pallido-thalamic circuit underlies the core symptoms of OCD, including unwanted, persistent, anxiety-provoking *obsessions* and repetitive, time-consuming *compulsions* (Berlim et al. 2008). This well-defined circuitry involves the DLPFC, or-

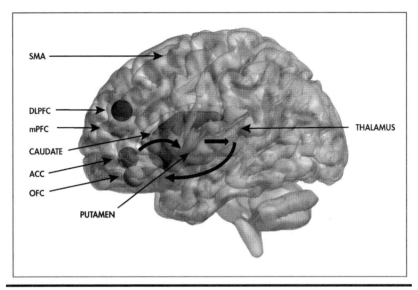

Figure 9–2. Obsessive-compulsive disorder (OCD) circuit.

See Plate 2 to view this figure in color.

Left-sided lateral view of the brain with medial structures also visible. Evidence suggests that the orbitofronto-striato-pallido-thalamic circuit underlies the core symptoms of OCD. This well-defined circuitry involves the dorsolateral prefrontal cortex (DLPFC), orbitofrontal cortex (OFC), medial prefrontal cortex (mPFC), anterior cingulate cortex (ACC), supplementary motor area (SMA), and basal ganglia, composed of the caudate and putamen (Del Casale et al. 2011). Image was visualized with the BrainNet Viewer (Xia et al. 2013).

bitofrontal cortex, medial prefrontal cortex, anterior cingulate gyrus, supplementary motor area, and basal ganglia (Del Casale et al. 2011; see Figure 9–2). All of these network "nodes" are potential targets for TMS, and many have been directly investigated with variable and sometimes conflicting results.

One of the earliest studies of TMS in treating OCD (Greenberg et al. 1997) suggested that high-frequency stimulation over both the left and right DLPFCs could reduce compulsive symptoms, but a later study (Sachdev et al. 2007) did not corroborate this finding. The active and sham groups did not differ on change in Yale-Brown Obsessive Compulsive Scale (Y-BOCS) or Maudsley Obsessive-Compulsive Inventory scores over 10 sessions, with or without correction for depression ratings. Over 20 sessions, there was a significant reduction in total Y-BOCS scores but not after controlling for depression. In general, high-frequency TMS protocols and DLPFC stimulation do not appear to be effective. There is evidence to suggest possible benefit from slow-frequency 1-Hz stimulation over the orbitofrontal cortex or supplementary motor area (Berlim et al. 2013); this may be explained by the inhibitory effects of low-frequency TMS on hyperactive orbitofronto-striatal circuits (Menzies et al. 2008).

At this time, there is insufficient evidence to confidently support the use of TMS in the treatment of OCD (Slotema et al. 2010) with figure-eight and other currently available TMS coils. New coil designs may be capable of stimulating the relevant circuits to ameliorate symptoms of OCD.

One study used an H coil (HAC or H7 coil) designed to target the medial prefrontal cortices and anterior cingulate cortices bilaterally in 41 patients with treatment-resistant OCD with moderate to severe symptoms. Treatments were administered after the patient's individual symptoms were provoked, and electroencephalogram measurements during a Stroop task were utilized to assess changes in error-related activity. Improvements were measured using the Y-BOCS. Initially, the study had four arms, a high-frequency arm of 20 Hz, a sham 20-Hz arm, a low-frequency arm of 1 Hz, and a sham 1-Hz arm. During the interim analysis, there was no difference between the sham and 1-Hz arms, so the study was continued with just 20-Hz high-frequency and sham arms. At the end of the study, the response rate in the 20-Hz arm was much greater than in the sham group, and the improvements lasted for a month after treatments ended. Interestingly, the improvement in the high-frequency group correlated with an increase in error-related negativity during the Stroop task following the treatment, suggesting that the improvement is related to the ability of the H7 coil to modify activity in the anterior cingulate (Carmi et al. 2015; Zangen et al. 2016).

Posttraumatic Stress Disorder

PTSD is characterized by a learned fear (due to a past traumatic event) that becomes generalized (Mahan and Ressler 2012). Fear conditioning and its circuitry are well conserved across vertebrate species, with the limbic system being the center of fear and emotion processing in humans and animals. Altered activity in the limbic regions of the amygdala, hippocampus, and prefrontal cortex is demonstrated in patients with PTSD (Karsen et al. 2014; Mahan and Ressler 2012; see Figure 9–3).

Given the success of targeting the DLPFC for depression, most studies also target this region for PTSD. A review by Karsen et al. (2014) included eight small studies ($N=133$) in which the TMS sites were either the left, right, or both DLPFCs or the bilateral medial prefrontal cortices. No statistically significant effect size was found, however, possibly because of the small sample sizes. Of the targets assessed, there was a trend

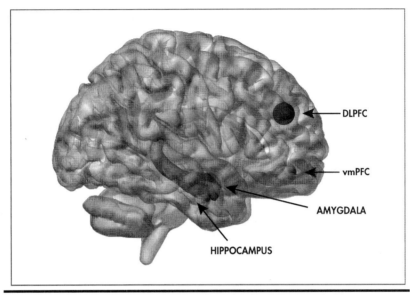

Figure 9–3. Posttraumatic stress disorder (PTSD) circuit.

See Plate 3 to view this figure in color.

Right-sided lateral view of structures implicated in PTSD. Functional neuroimaging findings in PTSD support the hypothesis that the amygdala is hyperresponsive, and ventral portions of medial prefrontal cortex (vmPFC) and right dorsolateral prefrontal cortex are hyporesponsive. Hippocampal volume and function appear to be abnormal as well. Image was visualized with the BrainNet Viewer (Xia et al. 2013).

toward efficacy when stimulating the right DLPFC at low frequency with a greater total number of stimuli/pulses (Karsen et al. 2014).

At this time, TMS treatment of PTSD remains experimental. Because many patients with PTSD also suffer from major depressive disorder, many will qualify for TMS therapy based on their mood disorder diagnosis and may also experience improvement in PTSD symptoms. Military veterans with combat- or operation-related PTSD may be referred to Department of Defense or Department of Veterans Affairs TMS research trials.

Addiction

Behaviors associated with addiction are complex and include preoccupation, craving, anticipation, bingeing, satiation, cessation, and withdrawal. The brain regions underlying each of these behaviors likely exert interconnected effects, working in concert to modulate different stages of the disorder (Koob and Volkow 2010). This results in a breadth of potential cortical targets for TMS therapy.

In a randomized controlled trial, Dinur-Klein et al. (2014) used deep TMS bilaterally over the lateral prefrontal and insular cortices to augment smoking cessation. A standard figure-eight TMS coil is unable to induce direct stimulation of deeper cortical areas, but using a specific H coil allows induction of a deeper electromagnetic field (see Chapter 10, "Current FDA-Cleared TMS Systems and Future Innovations in TMS Therapy"). In this study, 10 daily sessions of high-frequency deep TMS with an H-coil system reduced cigarette consumption, with the effect being most pronounced when treatment was applied following presentation of a smoking cue.

To date, the most common target for the treatment of addiction disorders is the left DLPFC at frequencies of 10–20 Hz (Grall-Bronnec and Sauvaget 2014; see Figure 9–4). A review of 18 studies involving approximately 400 patients with a variety of addictions, including nicotine, alcohol, recreational drugs, and food, suggests a role for TMS in reduction of craving (Grall-Bronnec and Sauvaget 2014). Assessment of these results needs to take into account the behavioral differences involved in these addictions; the significant heterogeneity in design, type, and target of TMS; and differences in final outcome measures across the 18 studies.

Chronic Pain

Pain perception is a multidimensional experience involving a widespread network of brain regions. Anatomical, electrophysiological, and functional imaging approaches have established the cortical areas that contribute to the perception of pain and that may be potential TMS targets for the treatment of chronic pain. A general conceptual framework divides the nociceptive network into lateral and medial components, which contribute to the sensory-discriminative and affective-motivational dimensions of pain, respectively (Melzack and Casey 1968). The cortical targets of the lateral system, involving afferent projections from the lateral thalamic nuclei, are mainly the primary and secondary somatosensory cortices. By contrast, the insula and anterior cingulate cortex are the main targets of the medial system and involve medial thalamic nuclei. In reality, pain processing is more complex. Connections exist between the cortical areas that receive direct nociceptive input and other cortical or subcortical brain regions (e.g., prefrontal cortex, motor cortex, periaqueductal gray matter) and are implicated in the cognitive-evaluative aspects of pain, pain modulation, and the integration of pain with other sensory modalities (Treede and Apkarian 2009; Vogt and Sikes 2009; see

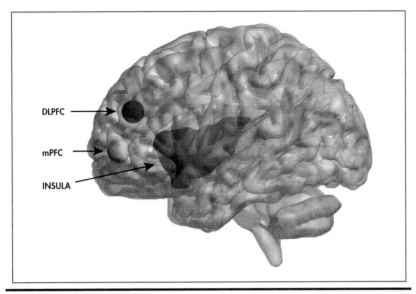

Figure 9–4. Addiction circuit.

See Plate 4 to view this figure in color.

Left-sided lateral view of potential transcranial magnetic stimulation (TMS) targets for addiction therapy. Damage to the insula has been associated with an increased ability to stop smoking, whereas cue activation of the medial prefrontal cortex (mPFC) has been seen in alcoholic patients. The most common target to date is the left dorsolateral prefrontal cortex (DLPFC), where TMS may have a role in craving reduction. The DLPFC has been studied in patients for a variety of addictions, including nicotine, alcohol, recreational drugs, and food. Image was visualized with the BrainNet Viewer (Xia et al. 2013).

Figure 9–5). It is now well established that structural and functional abnormalities are evident in these brain areas across numerous chronic pain conditions (Davis and Moayedi 2013).

TMS has been studied as a potential treatment for a variety of chronic pain syndromes, including fibromyalgia, neuropathic pain, facial pain, migraine, and irritable bowel syndrome, with several studies reporting significant pain reduction compared with sham treatment (Galhardoni et al. 2015). In general, high-frequency (10- or 20-Hz) stimulation to the primary motor cortex (M1) has yielded positive results (Johnson et al. 2006; Khedr et al. 2005; Lefaucheur et al. 2001; Pleger et al. 2004; Rollnik et al. 2002). The mechanism of action of M1 stimulation is not entirely understood, but there is reason to believe its analgesic effects rely on endogenous opioid systems (de Andrade et al. 2011). Some analgesic effects are also reported with high-frequency DLPFC stimulation in patients with phantom limb pain and fibromyalgia (Ahmed et al. 2011; Brighina et al. 2004; Short et al. 2011), but these effects likely involve a different

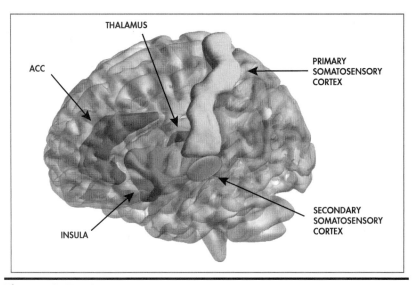

Figure 9–5.   Pain circuit.

See Plate 5 to view this figure in color.

Left-sided view of both lateral and medial structures involved in chronic pain. Pain processing is complex; however, a general conceptual framework has been adopted in which the structures involved are divided into lateral and medial components, which contribute to the sensory-discriminative and affective-motivational dimensions of pain, respectively. The lateral system includes the primary and secondary somatosensory cortices, whereas the insula and anterior cingulate cortex (ACC) are the main targets of the medial system. The thalamus plays a processing role in both systems. Image was visualized with the BrainNet Viewer (Xia et al. 2013).

mechanism (de Andrade et al. 2011). For both motor cortex and DLPFC stimulation, there is evidence to suggest that the analgesic effect depends on trans-synaptic stimulation of distant brain areas involved in pain integration and modulation (Hasan et al. 2014). For example, in an animal model, M1 stimulation resulted in decreased thalamic activity bilaterally and increased periaqueductal gray activity (França et al. 2013; Pagano et al. 2012). Moreover, the precise region of stimulation within these broad brain areas may have different effects. For example, homotopic analgesia (i.e., analgesia corresponding to the body part associated with a specific region of cortex) is observed with electrical transdural M1 stimulation in rats (Maarrawi et al. 2007).

Dementia

Dementia is a worldwide public health problem. The number of cases is expected to exceed 65 million by 2030 and is likely to double by 2050 (Rutherford et al. 2013). Alzheimer's disease (AD) accounts for more than half of all cases of dementia. Current drug treatments are of limited and temporary benefit.

Reports of TMS improving cognitive function began to emerge shortly after its introduction as a research tool. Over 60 studies with normally functioning, healthy subjects have reported significant improvement in speed and accuracy in a variety of tasks involving perceptual, motor, and executive processing (Luber and Lisanby 2014). In addition, a number of studies have specifically investigated TMS as a treatment for AD (Guerra et al. 2011) and other forms of dementia, including dementia with Lewy bodies (Liang et al. 2010) and vascular dementia (Pennisi et al. 2011).

High-frequency bilateral DLPFC stimulation has been shown to improve the accuracy of action naming and object naming in moderate to severe AD (Cotelli et al. 2008). Episodic memory and information processing speed have also been shown to improve following high-frequency TMS to the left DLPFC in patients with AD (Haffen et al. 2012).

High-frequency repetitive TMS has also been combined with cognitive training (rTMS-COG) using a proprietary medical device, the NeuroAD System (Neuronix, Yokneam, Israel). A prospective, randomized, double-blind, placebo-controlled study (Rabey et al. 2013) included 27 patients with AD (18 and 8 in the treatment and sham groups, respectively, and 1 dropout). The participants were categorized into groups with mild AD (Mini-Mental State Examination [MMSE] score=21–26) or moderate AD (MMSE score=18–20). The rTMS protocols were configured for six cortical areas (both dorsolateral prefrontal and parietal somatosensory association cortices and Broca's and Wernicke's areas). Patients received 10-Hz TMS at 90%–110% intensity for 5 days/week for 6 weeks. Neuropsychological assessments were performed using the Alzheimer's Disease Assessment Scale Cognitive subscale (ADAS-Cog), Clinical Global Impression of Change (CGIC) Scale, and MMSE before, immediately after, and 6 weeks after the end of rTMS-COG treatment. Significant improvement in cognition was observed among the patients with AD. Mean ADAS-Cog scores among those with mild AD improved by 5.46 points, which is remarkable considering that cholinesterase inhibitors result in an average improvement of 1.8 points over 12 weeks (Lee et al. 2015) and 2.7 points over 6 months (Birks 2006).

The NeuroAD System with its associated treatment protocol (stimulation of multiple cortical areas combined with cognitive training) is commercially available in Europe but is still considered investigational in the United States as of this writing. Although TMS is not a cure, it does appear to modify disease progression and may represent an important advance in AD treatment.

Other Disorders

Craving not only is a characteristic feature of addiction disorders but also plays a prominent role in *bulimia nervosa* and other conditions involving bingeing behaviors. Similar patterns of activation have been identified in addiction and obesity (Van den Eynde et al. 2010). High-frequency stimulation over the DLPFC may reduce these cravings or inhibit their development altogether (Uher et al. 2005), although whether this translates to reduced consumption has not yet been studied.

Previous studies of *autism spectrum disorder* have suggested a morphological disturbance resulting in a deficit of inhibition that leads patients with autism to process information excessively and be unable to successfully differentiate between target and irrelevant stimuli (Sokhadze et al. 2009). This lack of inhibition suggests a possible role for low-frequency TMS. For example, when assessed in combination with measured event-related potentials, low-frequency TMS minimized early cortical responses to irrelevant stimuli and increased responses to relevant stimuli (Sokhadze et al. 2010).

Other neurological disorders currently under study are those that have an associated motor aspect. These include Tourette syndrome, Parkinson's disease, epilepsy, multiple sclerosis, and traumatic brain injury. Research is also under way involving treatment of migraine and dystonia and rehabilitation following stroke.

Conclusion

Much research is still needed to discover various potential uses of TMS. Before successful TMS treatments can be developed, relevant neural circuitry of a disorder of interest must be understood. Once this circuitry is identified, we can then target the regions involved. The details of how TMS exerts its therapeutic effects are still unclear. Further investigation is needed to understand how TMS affects neural circuitry through long-term potentiation and long-term depression. This can be achieved with careful symptom and behavioral assessment and further augmented with the addition of neuroimaging (e.g., functional magnetic resonance imaging, positron emission tomography) and other techniques. Finally, a relatively unexplored use of TMS may be as a means to improve diagnostic methods and/or identify subtypes of disease. For example, the ability of TMS to create temporary and reversible disruptions in normal neuronal activity ("virtual lesions") on demand could serve as a diagnostic testing mechanism that psychiatry currently lacks.

KEY CLINICAL POINTS

- At this time, TMS has been cleared by the U.S. Food and Drug Administration for adult patients with major depression who have not responded to one or more antidepressant medications. All other uses are considered experimental or off-label and are not generally covered by health insurance.

- There is evidence from randomized controlled studies and meta-analyses to support the off-label use of TMS in the treatment of refractory negative symptoms of schizophrenia.

- Evidence from several open-label studies and one randomized controlled study suggests that a modified form of TMS combined with cognitive training may slow the cognitive decline of patients with mild to moderate Alzheimer's disease.

- There is insufficient evidence to support the off-label use of TMS in obsessive-compulsive disorder, posttraumatic stress disorder, and other conditions, but ongoing research and new technological developments may yield new insights and opportunities.

References

Ahmed MA, Mohamed SA, Sayed D: Long-term antalgic effects of repetitive transcranial magnetic stimulation of motor cortex and serum beta-endorphin in patients with phantom pain. Neurol Res 33(9):953–958, 2011 22080997

Berlim MT, Fleck MP, Turecki G: Current trends in the assessment and somatic treatment of resistant/refractory major depression: an overview. Ann Med 40(2):149–159, 2008 18293145

Berlim MT, Neufeld NH, Van den Eynde F: Repetitive transcranial magnetic stimulation (rTMS) for obsessive-compulsive disorder (OCD): an exploratory meta-analysis of randomized and sham-controlled trials. J Psychiatr Res 47(8):999–1006, 2013 23615189

Birks J: Cholinesterase inhibitors for Alzheimer's disease. Cochrane Database Syst Rev (1):CD005593, 2006 16437532

Brighina F, Piazza A, Vitello G, et al: rTMS of the prefrontal cortex in the treatment of chronic migraine: a pilot study. J Neurol Sci 227(1):67–71, 2004 15546593

Carmi L, Alyagon U, DAR R, et at: Deep transcranial magnetic stimulation (TMS) in obsessive compulsive disorder (OCD) patients. Eur Psychiatry 30 (suppl 1):794 2015

Cole JC, Green Bernacki C, Helmer A, et al: Efficacy of transcranial magnetic stimulation (TMS) in the treatment of schizophrenia: a review of the literature to date. Innov Clin Neurosci 12(7–8):12–19, 2015 26351619

Cotelli M, Manenti R, Cappa SF, et al: Transcranial magnetic stimulation improves naming in Alzheimer disease patients at different stages of cognitive decline. Eur J Neurol 15(12):1286–1292, 2008 19049544

Davis KD, Moayedi M: Central mechanisms of pain revealed through functional and structural MRI. J Neuroimmune Pharmacol 8(3):518–534, 2013 22825710

de Andrade DC, Mhalla A, Adam F, et al: Neuropharmacological basis of rTMS-induced analgesia: the role of endogenous opioids. Pain 152(2):320–326, 2011 21146300

Del Casale A, Kotzalidis GD, Rapinesi C, et al: Functional neuroimaging in obsessive-compulsive disorder. Neuropsychobiology 64(2):61–85, 2011 21701225

Dinur-Klein L, Dannon P, Hadar A, et al: Smoking cessation induced by deep repetitive transcranial magnetic stimulation of the prefrontal and insular cortices: a prospective, randomized controlled trial. Biol Psychiatry 76(9):742–749, 2014 25038985

Fitzgerald PB, Benitez J, Daskalakis JZ, et al: The treatment of recurring auditory hallucinations in schizophrenia with rTMS. World J Biol Psychiatry 7(2):119–122, 2006 16684685

França NR, Toniolo EF, Franciosi AC, et al: Antinociception induced by motor cortex stimulation: somatotopy of behavioral response and profile of neuronal activation. Behav Brain Res 250:211–221, 2013 23692698

Galhardoni R, Correia GS, Araujo H, et al: Repetitive transcranial magnetic stimulation in chronic pain: a review of the literature. Arch Phys Med Rehabil 96 (4 suppl):S156–S172, 2015 25437106

Grall-Bronnec M, Sauvaget A: The use of repetitive transcranial magnetic stimulation for modulating craving and addictive behaviours: a critical literature review of efficacy, technical and methodological considerations. Neurosci Biobehav Rev 47:592–613, 2014 25454360

Greenberg B, George MS, Martin JD, et al: Effect of prefrontal repetitive transcranial magnetic stimulation in obsessive-compulsive disorder: a preliminary study. Am J Psychiatry 154(6):867–869, 1997 9167520

Guerra A, Assenza F, Bressi F, et al: Transcranial magnetic stimulation studies in Alzheimer's disease. Int J Alzheimers Dis 2011:263817, 2011 21760985

Haffen E, Chopard G, Pretalli JB, et al: A case report of daily left prefrontal repetitive transcranial magnetic stimulation (rTMS) as an adjunctive treatment for Alzheimer disease. Brain Stimulat 5(3):264–266, 2012 22037125

Hasan M, Whiteley J, Bresnahan R, et al: Somatosensory change and pain relief induced by repetitive transcranial magnetic stimulation in patients with central poststroke pain. Neuromodulation 17(8):731–736, discussion 736, 2014 24934719

Hoffman RE, Boutros NN, Berman RM, et al: Transcranial magnetic stimulation of left temporoparietal cortex in three patients reporting hallucinated "voices." Biol Psychiatry 46(1):130–132, 1999 10394483

Hoffman RE, Hawkins KA, Gueorguieva R, et al: Transcranial magnetic stimulation of left temporoparietal cortex and medication-resistant auditory hallucinations. Arch Gen Psychiatry 60(1):49–56, 2003 12511172

Johnson S, Summers J, Pridmore S: Changes to somatosensory detection and pain thresholds following high frequency repetitive TMS of the motor cortex in individuals suffering from chronic pain. Pain 123(1–2):187–192, 2006 16616419

Karsen EF, Watts BV, Holtzheimer PE: Review of the effectiveness of transcranial magnetic stimulation for post-traumatic stress disorder. Brain Stimulat 7(2):151–157, 2014 24486424

Khedr EM, Kotb H, Kamel NF, et al: Longlasting antalgic effects of daily sessions of repetitive transcranial magnetic stimulation in central and peripheral neuropathic pain. J Neurol Neurosurg Psychiatry 76(6):833–838, 2005 15897507

Koob GF, Volkow ND: Neurocircuitry of addiction. Neuropsychopharmacology 35(1):217–238, 2010 19710631

Lee JH, Hong YJ, Bae HJ, et al: The effects of galantamine treatment on attention and its relationship with cognition and activities of daily living in patients with mild to moderate Alzheimer's disease. J Clin Neurol 11(1):66–72, 2015 25628739

Lefaucheur JP, Drouot X, Nguyen JP: Interventional neurophysiology for pain control: duration of pain relief following repetitive transcranial magnetic stimulation of the motor cortex. Neurophysiol Clin 31(4):247–252, 2001 11601430

Liang X, Liu K, Guo L: Repetitive transcranial magnetic stimulation (rTMS): a possible novel therapeutic approach to dementia with Lewy bodies. Med Hypotheses 74(5):877–879, 2010 20006914

Luber B, Lisanby SH: Enhancement of human cognitive performance using transcranial magnetic stimulation (TMS). Neuroimage 85 (Pt 3):961–997, 2014 23770409

Maarrawi J, Peyron R, Mertens P, et al: Motor cortex stimulation for pain control induces changes in the endogenous opioid system. Neurology 69(9):827–834, 2007 17724284

Mahan AL, Ressler KJ: Fear conditioning, synaptic plasticity and the amygdala: implications for posttraumatic stress disorder. Trends Neurosci 35(1):24–35, 2012 21798604

Melzack R, Casey KL: Sensory, Motivational, and Central Control Determinants of Pain. Springfield, IL, Charles C Thomas, 1968

Menzies L, Chamberlain SR, Laird AR, et al: Integrating evidence from neuroimaging and neuropsychological studies of obsessive-compulsive disorder: the orbitofronto-striatal model revisited. Neurosci Biobehav Rev 32(3):525–549, 2008 18061263

Pagano RL, Fonoff ET, Dale CS, et al: Motor cortex stimulation inhibits thalamic sensory neurons and enhances activity of PAG neurons: possible pathways for antinociception. Pain 153(12):2359–2369, 2012 23017297

Pallanti S, Quercioli L: Treatment-refractory obsessive-compulsive disorder: methodological issues, operational definitions and therapeutic lines. Prog Neuropsychopharmacol Biol Psychiatry 30(3):400–412, 2006 16503369

Pennisi G, Ferri R, Cantone M, et al: A review of transcranial magnetic stimulation in vascular dementia. Dement Geriatr Cogn Disord 31(1):71–80, 2011 21242688

Pleger B, Janssen F, Schwenkreis P, et al: Repetitive transcranial magnetic stimulation of the motor cortex attenuates pain perception in complex regional pain syndrome type I. Neurosci Lett 356(2):87–90, 2004 14746870

Rabey JM, Dobronevsky E, Aichenbaum S, et al: Repetitive transcranial magnetic stimulation combined with cognitive training is a safe and effective modality for the treatment of Alzheimer's disease: a randomized, double-blind study. J Neural Transm (Vienna) 120(5):813–819, 2013 23076723

Rollnik JD, Wüstefeld S, Däuper J, et al: Repetitive transcranial magnetic stimulation for the treatment of chronic pain—a pilot study. Eur Neurol 48(1):6–10, 2002 12138303

Rutherford G, Gole R, Moussavi Z: rTMS as a treatment of Alzheimer's disease with and without comorbidity of depression: a review. Neurosci J 2013:679389, doi: 10.1155/2013/679389 2013 26317096

Sachdev PS, Loo CK, Mitchell PB, et al: Repetitive transcranial magnetic stimulation for the treatment of obsessive compulsive disorder: a double-blind controlled investigation. Psychol Med 37(11):1645–1649 2007 17655805

Short EB, Borckardt JJ, Anderson BS, et al: Ten sessions of adjunctive left prefrontal rTMS significantly reduces fibromyalgia pain: a randomized, controlled pilot study. Pain 152(11):2477–2484, 2011 21764215

Silbersweig DA, Stern E, Frith C, et al: A functional neuroanatomy of hallucinations in schizophrenia. Nature 378(6553):176–179, 1995 7477318

Slotema CW, Blom JD, Hoek HW, et al: Should we expand the toolbox of psychiatric treatment methods to include repetitive transcranial magnetic stimulation (rTMS)? A meta-analysis of the efficacy of rTMS in psychiatric disorders. J Clin Psychiatry 71(7):873–884, 2010 20361902

Slotema CW, Blom JD, van Lutterveld R, et al: Review of the efficacy of transcranial magnetic stimulation for auditory verbal hallucinations. Biol Psychiatry 76(2):101–110, 2014 24315551

Sokhadze EM, El-Baz A, Baruth J, et al: Effects of low frequency repetitive transcranial magnetic stimulation (rTMS) on gamma frequency oscillations and event-related potentials during processing of illusory figures in autism. J Autism Dev Disord 39(4):619–634, 2009 19030976

Sokhadze E, Baruth J, Tasman A, et al: Low-frequency repetitive transcranial magnetic stimulation (rTMS) affects event-related potential measures of novelty processing in autism. Appl Psychophysiol Biofeedback 35(2):147–161, 2010 19941058

Stanford AD, Corcoran C, Bulow P, et al: High-frequency prefrontal repetitive transcranial magnetic stimulation for the negative symptoms of schizophrenia: a case series. J ECT 27(1):11–17, 2011 20966771

Treede R, Apkarian A: Nociceptive Processing in the Cerebral Cortex. New York, Elsevier, 2009

Uher R, Yoganathan D, Mogg A, et al: Effect of left prefrontal repetitive transcranial magnetic stimulation on food craving. Biol Psychiatry 58(10):840–842, 2005 16084855

Van den Eynde F, Claudino AM, Mogg A, et al: Repetitive transcranial magnetic stimulation reduces cue-induced food craving in bulimic disorders. Biol Psychiatry 67(8):793–795, 2010 20060105

Vogt B, Sikes R: Cingulate Nociceptive Circuitry and Roles in Pain Processing: The Cingulate Premotor Pain Model. New York, Oxford University Press, 2009

Xia MR, Wang JH, HE Y: BrainNet Viewer: a network visualization tool for human brain connectomics. PLoS One 8(7):e68910, 2013 23861951

Zangen A, Carmi L, Alyagon U, et al: Deep transcranial magnetic stimulation of the anterior cingulate cortex in obsessive compulsive disorder patients. Brain Stimul 9(5):e4 2016

10

Current FDA-Cleared TMS Systems and Future Innovations in TMS Therapy

Ian A. Cook, M.D., DFAPA

Treating patients with transcranial magnetic stimulation (TMS) demands the use of a system that is capable of generating magnetic fields with the desired spatial and temporal characteristics to stimulate the intended brain structures. There are many ways to construct a TMS system that can meet those requirements, and in this chapter, I review some technologies that have been developed into clinically available products. Before I delve into these specifics, however, some consideration of the bigger picture is in order.

In the United States, TMS systems are among the medical devices regulated by the U.S. Food and Drug Administration (FDA), specifically by the Center for Devices and Radiological Health. The FDA reviews information provided by manufacturers of therapeutic medical products to assess their safety and efficacy in treating specific medical conditions. At the present time, there are five manufacturers with FDA clearance to market therapeutic TMS systems in the United States, all for use in treating depression. Patients and physicians in other countries may be able to use different TMS systems because each jurisdiction has its own rules and regulations regarding legal access to these medical devices.

Although the FDA may regulate how manufacturers make their products available in the United States, licensed physicians may practice medicine by using a product as intended ("on-label") or in alternative ways ("off-label") that are consistent with their understanding of the best ways to treat their own patients (i.e., the FDA "does not regulate the practice of medicine," per Wittich et al. [2012, p. 982]). A physician uses a product on-label by adhering to the written information regarding use, relying on instructions that the manufacturer has developed and the FDA has reviewed. Normally, this may include use for a specified clinical condition or indication and adhering to the specified dosing, as detailed in the "package insert" document that accompanies medications or the "instructions for use" manual that accompanies devices. Examples of an off-label use include prescribing a product to treat a different condition (e.g., using TMS to treat bipolar depression or tinnitus) and using different parameters (e.g., prescribing a medication dose that is outside the range in the package insert, providing TMS treatment at a frequency not in the "instructions for use" manual). The FDA bases its labeling decisions on the data that are provided for review. Therefore, the boundary between on-label and off-label use could reflect an absence of data (e.g., if no manufacturer has submitted studies using a 1-Hz repetition rate), or there could be data indicating the absence of a demonstrated effect (e.g., failed trials for treating some clinical condition, which would not be submitted for review).

The biomedical literature may describe findings of safety and effectiveness from encouraging research trials of TMS devices used in ways outside current labeling, but practitioners should remember that health care payers may have coverage policies that limit access for off-label TMS treatment. This is often a "moving target," with policies and restrictions that change, and inquiry ahead of treatment is important to determine what coverage policy may apply to a given patient at a given time.

This emphasis on dry regulatory considerations is relevant at the outset of this chapter for two reasons: First, it is important for clinicians to understand the tools they use (i.e., the tools' capabilities and where use crosses from on-label to off-label parameters). Second, to present reliable facts about the devices, I have derived much of the information on specific products from the legally reviewed documents the manufacturers submitted to the FDA, supplemented by information from the peer-reviewed medical literature. Some information in the remainder of this chapter concerns principles that are common to all the legally marketed devices, whereas other information may be unique to a particular system.

Contextual Notes From Foundational Biophysics

Regardless of manufacturer, all five current TMS systems rely on the principle of magnetic induction, first described by Michael Faraday in 1831 and independently (re)discovered by Joseph Henry in 1832. A common representation of Faraday's law, as part of the Maxwell-Faraday equation, states that a time-varying magnetic field will always accompany a spatially varying electrical field, and vice versa, expressed mathematically as

$$\nabla \times \mathbf{E} = -\frac{\partial \mathbf{B}}{\partial t}$$

where $\mathbf{E}$ is the electrical field, $\mathbf{B}$ is the magnetic field (both fields being functions of both position and time), and $\nabla \times \mathbf{E}$ denotes the curl vector field operator. In the context of clinical TMS systems, what this means is that *a changing magnetic field will generate an electrical field and a current* in a conductive medium, such as brain structures or scalp tissue.

When the electrical field and current are of sufficient magnitude, a neuron in the field will become depolarized and an action potential will propagate along its axon. Once a neuron has become depolarized and has "fired" with an action potential, it cannot fire again until its refractory period is over. Thus, there is a physiological limit to how fast the magnetic field can change to produce a series of distinct nerve impulses.

Because the neuronal depolarization phenomenon is nonlinear, a neuron does not fire more intensely if the stimulation is markedly larger than that needed to produce a depolarization rather than just minimally above threshold. Pragmatically, stimulating at levels in excess of the motor threshold does not make the specific neurons in the target region fire "harder," but it does serve to increase the volume in space in which the depolarization threshold is met or exceeded (and thus may cause additional, unintended brain circuits to be stimulated).

Design of TMS Systems

All the devices that have FDA clearance as TMS systems (as of February 2017) share at least two common elements:

- A coil to generate the time-varying magnetic field
- A microprocessor-controlled source of electrical energy

There are numerous approaches to coil design, such as variations in the size and shape of the coil and use of ferromagnetic materials (to alter the field properties) versus an air core design. The following coils are commercially available for clinical use as part of the cleared TMS systems:

- Figure-eight coil with a ferromagnetic core (Neuronetics)
- H coil (Hesed coil) with an air core (Brainsway)
- Figure-eight coil with an air core (Magstim, MagVenture, and Neurosoft)

Other coils, such as circular coils, are also available for research or other purposes. Coils can differ considerably in the electrical fields they induce. For example, a circular coil has maximum intensity in the tissue directly under the coil windings, whereas a figure-eight coil can be configured so that magnetic fields add at the crossing point of the "8," yielding a focal area of high intensity that can be "aimed" at specific neuroanatomical targets (Figure 10–1).

A comprehensive examination of the surface electrical field patterns with 50 coil designs was conducted by Deng et al. (2013) at Duke University. A comparison of the fields from an air core figure-eight coil, a ferromagnetic core figure-eight coil, and an H1 coil can be seen in Figure 10–2. Although visual inspection illustrates how different the patterns may be, the clinical relevance of these differences can best be assessed only through head-to-head trials, but such work has not yet been conducted.

It is noteworthy that heat is generated in the coils, in proportion to the resistance of the conductor and to the square of the current (i.e., I^2R

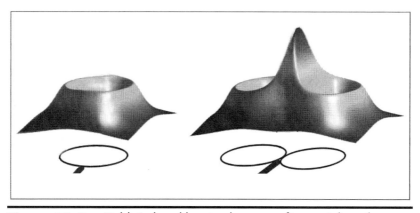

Figure 10–1.   Fields induced by circular versus figure-eight coils.

See Plate 6 to view this figure in color.

Electrical field intensity is displayed by both height and color.

Source.   Based on Cohen et al. 1990 and Thielscher and Kammer 2002.

heating losses). Dissipation of the heat produced in the coil is addressed in current products by passive air cooling, by forcing air to flow over the coil assembly, or by circulating a liquid coolant. Tales from the early days of TMS describe cooling the coils in buckets of ice water (M. George, personal communication, 2016).

The first report of a clinically useful TMS system is generally recognized as that by Anthony Barker and colleagues from the University of Sheffield in the United Kingdom (Barker et al. 1985). That device was initially developed as a diagnostic tool for performing neurological evaluations. Stimulation of the motor cortex with single magnetic pulses could elicit motor activity in terms of involuntary muscle contractions, and this system could also be used to interrogate the integrity of motor outflow tracts. Other uses soon followed, such as applying single pulses to produce a transient disruption in normal neuronal activity (a "virtual lesion") in order to study the physiology of normal and pathological brain function (see Pascual-Leone et al. 2000). Therapeutic use depended on the development of systems that could safely produce sustained trains of repetitive pulses, and the first case of psychiatric treatment with repetitive TMS (rTMS) was reported by Mark George and colleagues at the National Institute of Mental Health (George et al. 1995).

Although the sophistication of TMS systems has since evolved considerably, the fundamental elements of the electronics continued to consist of a means to store a large amount of electrical energy (e.g., a capacitor);

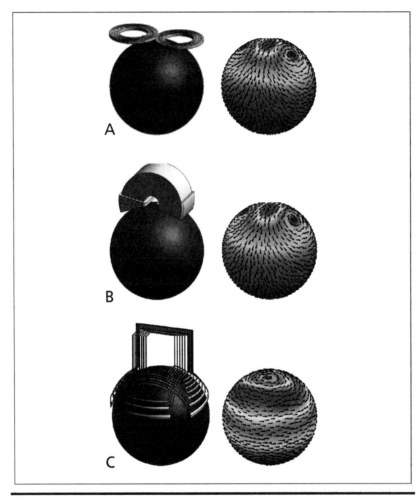

Figure 10–2.   Electrical fields from three example coil designs.

See Plate 7 to view this figure in color.
(A) Figure-eight coil, air core; (B) figure-eight coil, ferromagnetic core; and (C) H1 coil, air core.
Source.   Adapted from Deng et al. 2013.

a means to charge it; a means to discharge the energy rapidly through the coil; and a means to produce these pulses in a controlled, regular pattern (Cowey 2005). Contemporary designs employ microprocessor circuits to control the system and provide other useful features (e.g., for monitoring progress during a treatment session, for monitoring the temperature of the coil) instead of the analog circuits used initially.

TMS Devices With FDA Permission to Market in the United States

The FDA provides the following definition of an *rTMS system*:

> A repetitive transcranial magnetic stimulation system is an external device that delivers transcranial repetitive pulsed magnetic fields of sufficient magnitude to induce neural action potentials in the prefrontal cortex to treat the symptoms of major depressive disorder without inducing seizure in patients who have failed at least one antidepressant medication and are currently not on any antidepressant therapy (21 CFR 882.5805 [Code of Federal Regulations]).

This definition applies to all currently marketed rTMS products, categorized as Class II—special controls. By this definition, an rTMS system is not implanted; it induces action potentials without inducing a seizure, so it is distinct from devices for electroconvulsive therapy (ECT; covered in 21 CFR 882.5940); it targets the prefrontal cortex; it is intended for use in patients with major depressive disorder with at least one treatment failure; and it is intended to be used as stand-alone or monotherapy, as opposed to a treatment added onto pharmacotherapy. However, clinicians commonly use TMS as an adjunct for patients already prescribed psychotropic medication(s) (e.g., Carpenter et al. 2012).

Therapeutic TMS devices have been cleared for marketing in the United States via a so-called "510(k)" regulatory pathway. The regular 510(k) pathway allows for clearance for a low- to moderate-risk device for which there is "substantial equivalence" in safety and effectiveness to another lawfully marketed device (a "predicate" device); the de novo 510(k) pathway allows for approval of low- to moderate-risk devices for which general controls or general and special controls provide reasonable assurance of safety and effectiveness but for which there is no legally marketed predicate device.

NEURONETICS: NEUROSTAR TMS THERAPY SYSTEM

In late 2008, Neuronetics, Inc. (Malvern, Pennsylvania) was the first company to receive FDA clearance for a therapeutic TMS device, the NeuroStar TMS Therapy System. Table 10–1 summarizes the key parameters of the device, which is depicted in Figure 10–3. This system was approved in part on the basis of a pivotal trial, in which 301 adults who had not benefited from prior antidepressant medications were randomly assigned to active or sham treatment (Avery et al. 2008; Janicak et al. 2008; O'Reardon et al. 2007). Sessions were conducted five times/

Table 10–1. Description of the Neuronetics NeuroStar TMS Therapy System

Product name	NeuroStar TMS Therapy System
FDA status	510(k) de novo clearance K061053, October 2008
Related FDA actions	DEN070003, October 7, 2008
	K083538, December 16, 2008
	K130233, April 30, 2013
	K133408, March 28, 2014;
	K160703, June 10, 2016
	K161519, September 11, 2016
Coil	Biphasic figure-eight coil with ferromagnetic core
Pulse parameters approved	185-microsecond pulse width
	10-Hz repetition rate
	4-second train duration
	26-second intertrain interval
	3,000 pulses/session, over 37.5 minutes
Device capabilities	Repetition rate 0.1–30 Hz
	Magnetic field intensity 0.22–1.6 standard motor threshold units
	Train duration 1–20 seconds
	Intertrain interval 10–60 seconds
Elements of system, as described in FDA 510(k) filing	Mobile console with electronics
	Treatment coil
	Gantry that supports treatment coil
	Head support system with laser guidance
	SenStar Treatment link for contact sensing and monitoring magnetic field and surface field cancellation

Source. Information derived from U.S. Food and Drug Administration (FDA) filings (https://www.accessdata.fda.gov/cdrh_docs/pdf6/K061053.pdf).

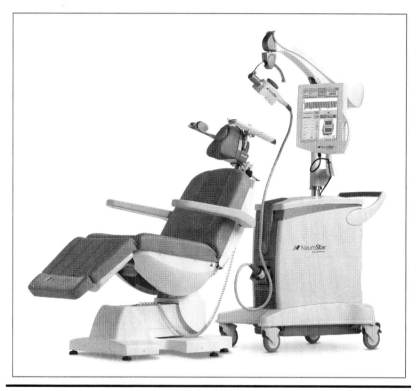

Figure 10–3.   NeuroStar TMS Therapy System.
Source.   Image courtesy of Neuronetics, Inc.

week with TMS at 10 pulses/second, 120% of motor threshold, and 3,000 pulses/session for 4–6 weeks. The primary outcome was the symptom score change as assessed at week 4 with the Montgomery-Åsberg Depression Rating Scale (MADRS); secondary outcomes included changes on the Hamilton Depression Rating Scale (HDRS) and response and remission rates with both scales.

The NeuroStar TMS Therapy System contains a number of patented features related to system design and user interface. A patented figure-eight coil with a ferromagnetic core is encased in a housing shaped to fit over the prefrontal area of the head—that is, over the target used in the pivotal trial—and is attached to a movable gantry with a gravity compensation mechanism. The use of an iron core promotes heat dissipation and eliminates the need for an external cooling system. It also increases the energy efficiency of magnetic field generation, with implications for the engineering design of the electronics that drives the coil. The shape of the coil housing may limit ease of use in stimulating brain regions other than the prefrontal cortex. The included treatment chair allows for multiple preprogrammed configurations related to height, degree of recline, and lumbar/leg support. The attached head support system can be adjusted for patient comfort and helps to prevent inadvertent head movement during treatment. Coil position is replicated from one treatment session to another using a built-in system of coordinates. The SenStar Treatment Link serves as a patient interface and performs several functions, including contact sensing and magnetic field detection. The MT Assist proprietary clinical software implements an algorithm to assist the operator in determining the motor threshold. The touch screen monitor allows entry of individual patient treatment parameters, coil position, and chair settings for future recall. The monitor also provides visual feedback to the operator regarding coil contact and alignment as well as real-time reporting of each treatment session, including elapsed time and number of pulses delivered.

The introduction of this system in 2008 was followed by critical work securing appropriate Current Procedural Terminology codes from the American Medical Association for demonstrating use of TMS procedures, which then facilitated the writing of coverage policies for TMS treatment by health care payers.

In a subsequent FDA 510(k) approval action, the stimulation parameters for on-label use were modified to allow for an intertrain interval (ITI) of between 11 and 26 seconds. Using the standard pulse train duration of 4 seconds, the new ITI changes the minimum cycle time from 30 seconds to 15 seconds, and thus the time for a 3,000-pulse treatment changes from 37.5 minutes to 18.75 minutes. It appears likely that other manufacturers may also seek 510(k) approvals for this change in ITI.

BRAINSWAY: DEEP TMS SYSTEM

The second product to receive FDA clearance as a therapeutic TMS device was the Deep TMS System from Brainsway, Inc. (Jerusalem, Israel, and Hackensack, New Jersey), cleared in early 2013. Table 10–2 summarizes the key parameters of the Brainsway Deep TMS System, depicted in Figure 10–4. This device uses a different coil design intended to produce deeper stimulation (see below) and also different stimulation parameters from the Neuronetics device; it was approved in part on the basis of a pivotal randomized clinical trial (Levkovitz et al. 2015) that recruited 212 adults with major depression. Twenty sessions of deep TMS at 18 Hz over the prefrontal cortex were administered for 4 weeks, and then sessions continued biweekly for 12 weeks. The pri-

Table 10–2. Description of the Brainsway Deep TMS System

Product name	Brainsway Deep TMS System
FDA status	510(k) clearance K122288, January 7, 2013
Coil	H coil with air core, air cooling
Pulse parameters approved	370-microsecond pulse width
	18-Hz repetition rate
	2-second train duration
	20-second intertrain interval
	1,980 pulses/session, over 20.1 minutes
Device capabilities	Repetition rate 0.02–30 Hz
	Magnetic field intensity 0.6–1.4 standard motor threshold units
	Train duration 1–20 seconds
	Intertrain interval 10–60 seconds
Elements of system, as described in FDA 510(k) filing	TMS neurostimulator
	Electromagnetic coil (H1)
	Cooling system
	Positioning system

Source. Information derived from U.S. Food and Drug Administration (FDA) filings (https://www.fda.gov/cdrh/510k/K122288.pdf)).

mary outcome measure was the change in the HDRS score, and the secondary outcome measures were response and remission rates at week 5.

The Deep TMS System also has a uniquely designed treatment coil. The Hesed H1 coil is contained within a helmet-like housing that fits over the patient's head. Coil windings run tangential to the head in a unique pattern and provide convergent electrical fields from various directions (Roth et al. 2002). This coil design is intended to produce an electrical field that can depolarize neurons at a greater depth but with a more diffuse field than is possible with devices using the figure-eight coil. With this system, treatment parameters are entered using a dial and touch screen. A monitor provides real-time reporting of each treatment session, including elapsed time and number of pulses delivered. The patient sits in an upright position, and any comfortable chair may be used.

Brainsway has developed a series of unique coil designs, each intended to concentrate the magnetic field toward particular anatomical

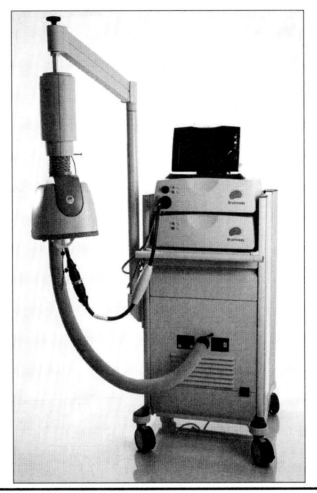

Figure 10–4. Brainsway Deep TMS System.

Source. Image courtesy of Brainsway, Inc.

targets (e.g., bilateral prefrontal cortices, primary motor cortex) (Advanced Mental Health Care 2012). At present, only the H1 coil is cleared by the FDA for clinical use, and other designs are investigational products at this time. This system is also unique in receiving FDA clearance based on a trial that used 18-Hz stimulation and treatment sessions comprising 1,980 pulses in 20.1 minutes; in contrast, the other four TMS systems detailed in this chapter were initially cleared based on data with 10-Hz stimulation and 3,000 pulses in 37.5 minutes, as in the original pivotal trial by Neuronetics (O'Reardon et al. 2007). The FDA's recent revisions to allow 3,000 pulses at 10 Hz to be delivered in 18.75 minutes (ITI=11 seconds) has reduced this differentiation.

MAGSTIM: RAPID^2 THERAPY SYSTEM

In 2015, the third rTMS therapeutic system to receive FDA clearance was the Rapid^2 Therapy System from the Magstim Company, Ltd. (Whitland, United Kingdom, and Morrisville, North Carolina). Of note, this company received clearance for a single-pulse TMS stimulator device for peripheral nerve stimulation use in 2000 (K992911) and historically traces its corporate lineage to Novametrix Medical Systems, the company that sought to commercialize the original work by A. Barker, I. L.Freeston, R. Jalinous, and M. Polson at the University of Sheffield in the 1980s (see https://www.magstim.com/heritage); many of the clinical studies prior to the NeuroStar system's clearance were done using Magstim equipment. Table 10–3 summarizes the key parameters of this device, which is shown in Figure 10–5. This device was cleared on the basis of substantial equivalency to the NeuroStar system without an additional clinical trial.

A figure-eight coil with an air-cooled system is used for treatment and is attached to an articulated stand without gravity compensation. Multiple pulse frequencies are possible. An optional lightweight, handheld coil is available for use in motor threshold determination; pulses can be triggered by a push-button switch on the coil unit. Coil position is replicated from one treatment to another by using a cap marked to show coil location or some other method such as an electroencephalographic montage net placed on the patient's head. An optional adjustable chair with headrest is available. Treatment parameters are entered using a dial and touch screen; storage of individual patient treatment parameters is not possible with current software (as of early 2017). The computer display provides real-time reporting of the parameters of each treatment session, including elapsed time and number of pulses delivered. Contact sensing is not available. In addition to the standard figure-eight coil that was cleared by the FDA for therapeutic use, other coil designs are available to allow flexibility for research purposes.

MAGVENTURE: MAGVITA TMS THERAPY SYSTEM

The fourth TMS system with FDA clearance (awarded July 2015) is the MagVita TMS Therapy System from MagVenture A/S (Farum, Denmark, and Alpharetta, Georgia). MagVenture's sibling company, Tonica Elektronik A/S, received FDA clearance for peripheral nerve magnetic

Table 10–3. Description of the Magstim Rapid^2 Therapy System

Product name	Rapid^2 Therapy System
FDA status Related FDA actions	510(k) clearance K143531, May 8, 2015
Related FDA actions	K162935, March 10, 2017
Coil	Biphasic figure-eight coil, air core, air cooling
Pulse parameters approved	300-microsecond pulse width
	10-Hz repetition rate
	4-second train duration
	26-second intertrain interval
	3,000 pulses/session, over 37.5 minutes
Device capabilities	Repetition rate 0.1–30 Hz
	Magnetic field intensity 0.28–1.9 standard motor threshold units
	Train duration 1–20 seconds
	Intertrain interval 10–60 seconds
Elements of system, as described in FDA 510(k) filing	User interface
	Mainframe
	Power supply
	Air film coil
	Coil stand
	Accessory foot switch

Source.   Information derived from U.S. Food and Drug Administration (FDA) filings (https://www.accessdata.fda.gov/cdrh_docs/pdf14/K143531.pdf).

stimulators in 1993 (K926516, to Dantec Medical, their U.S. affiliate), but this was for use as a diagnostic tool only. Table 10–4 summarizes the key parameters of this device, which is shown in Figure 10–6. This device was cleared on the basis of substantial equivalency to the NeuroStar system without an additional clinical trial.

The MagVita system employs a liquid cooling system to ensure operation within expected parameters during prolonged usage. The coil is attached to an articulated arm without gravity compensation, and a handheld coil is available for use in determining the motor threshold. An optional adjustable chair is available; it employs a special pillow de-

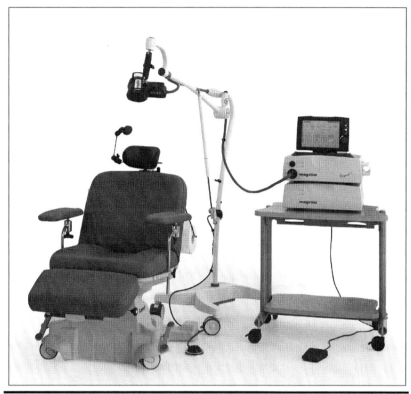

Figure 10–5. Magstim Rapid² Therapy System.

Source.   Image courtesy of Magstim Company, Ltd.

signed to limit head movement. Coil position is replicated from one treatment session to another by using a cap marked to show coil location or some other method such as an electroencephalographic montage net placed on the patient's head; contact sensing is not available. Treatment parameters are entered using a dial and touch screen; storage of individual patient parameters is not possible. In addition to the figure-eight coil that was cleared by the FDA as part of the therapeutic system, other coils are available to provide flexibility in the research setting.

NEUROSOFT: NEUROSOFT TMS SYSTEM

The fifth TMS system with FDA clearance (awarded December 2016) is the Neurosoft TMS System from Neurosoft (Ivanovo, Russia; distributed in the United States by Caputron Medical, New York, New York). Table 10–5 summarizes the key parameters of this device, which is

Table 10–4. Description of the MagVenture MagVita TMS Therapy System

Product name	MagVita TMS Therapy System
FDA status	510(k) clearance K150641, July 31, 2015
Related FDA actions	K170114, May 1, 2017
Coil	Figure-eight coil, air core, liquid cooling
Pulse parameters approved	290-microsecond pulse width
	10-Hz repetition rate
	4-second train duration
	26-second intertrain interval
	3,000 pulses/session, over 37.5 minutes
Device capabilities	Repetition rate 0.1–30 Hz (0.1–100 Hz depending on model)
	Magnetic field intensity 0–1.7 standard motor threshold units
Elements of system, as described in FDA 510(k) filing	MagPro stimulator and trolley
	Coil C-B60 for motor threshold determination
	Coil Cool-B65 for treatment with coil cooler unit
	Treatment chair
	Vacuum pump with vacuum pillow
	Flexible arm mounted on trolley

Source. Information derived from U.S. Food and Drug Administration (FDA) filings (https://www.accessdata.fda.gov/cdrh_docs/pdf15/k150641.pdf).

shown in Figure 10–7. This device was cleared on the basis of substantial equivalency to the Magstim and MagVenture systems as predicate devices, without an additional clinical trial. The system employs a liquid cooling system to ensure operation within expected parameters during prolonged usage. The coil is attached to an articulated arm without gravity compensation.

Vignettes

Three anecdotal vignettes are provided to illustrate the clinical use of these TMS systems. It must be emphasized that there are no published

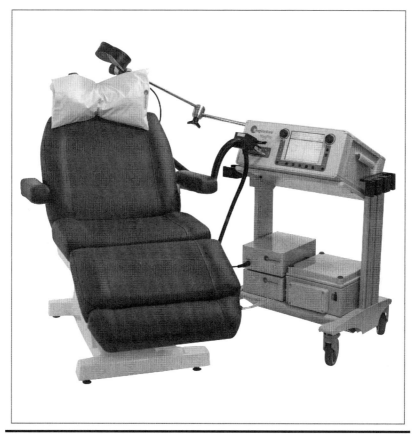

Figure 10–6. MagVita TMS Therapy System.

Source.   Image courtesy of MagVenture A/S.

comparative head-to-head effectiveness studies to provide systematic evidence comparing and contrasting treatment with the different systems. Some of the details of the following case vignettes have been altered to respect patient confidentiality and privacy.

CLINICAL VIGNETTE

The patient is a 48-year-old woman who had tried over five different antidepressant treatment regimens (monotherapies and combinations) at adequate doses and durations, as well as a course of cognitive-behavioral therapy, all in the current episode. The patient took medical leave from her employer—because of her depression, she was unable to perform her usual job responsibilities—and she was nearing the end of her paid leave period. TMS was a covered benefit under her health insurance policy, and she was referred by her treating psychiatrist to a TMS program.

Table 10–5.　Description of the Neurosoft TMS System

Product name	Neurosoft TMS System
FDA status	510(k) clearance K160309, December 22, 2016
Coil	Figure-eight coil, air core, liquid cooling
Pulse parameters approved	280-microsecond pulse width
	10-Hz repetition rate
	4-second train duration
	26-second intertrain interval
	3,000 pulses/session, over 37.5 minutes
Device capabilities	Repetition rate 0.1–30 Hz (100 Hz with additional PC controller)
	Pulse train duration 0.5–100 seconds
	Magnetic field intensity 0–2.39 standard motor threshold units
Elements of system, as described in FDA 510(k) filing	Stimulator, cooling unit, power unit, and trolley
	Flexible arm for coil positioning and coil holder
	Coil FEC-02-100-C for motor threshold determination
	Coil AFEC-02-100-C

Source. Information derived from U.S. Food and Drug Administration (FDA) filings (https://www.accessdata.fda.gov/cdrh_docs/pdf16/K160309.pdf).

She was evaluated and found to be an appropriate candidate for treatment; she had no prior TMS experience. After discussion with her treating psychiatrist, she began TMS while continuing to take a selective serotonin reuptake inhibitor antidepressant augmented with a second-generation antipsychotic, having voiced a strong preference to continue these agents while receiving TMS "just in case they were helping me more than was apparent." Treatment was initiated using 3,000 pulses/session at 10 Hz, administered over the dorsolateral prefrontal cortex (DLPFC) target assessed at the F3 electrode site with a system employing a figure-eight coil. Symptoms were monitored weekly with the 30-item Inventory of Depressive Symptomatology—Self-Report (IDS-SR30) and the 9-item Patient Health Questionnaire (PHQ-9). The patient noted

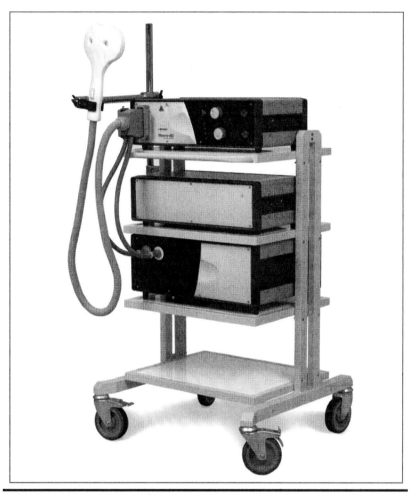

Figure 10–7. Neurosoft TMS System.

Source.   Image courtesy of Neurosoft/Caputron Medical.

symptom improvement in several domains after 10 sessions and further improvement after 20 sessions, and she was in remission around treatment 30. She then received six more tapering treatments, as had been done in the O'Reardon et al. (2007) trial, and was returned to the care of her treating psychiatrist. She was given copies of the IDS-SR30 and PHQ-9 for continued self-monitoring. For continuity of care, the TMS physician contacted the patient's treating psychiatrist by telephone to clarify the psychiatrist's understanding of TMS, discuss the empiric desirability of not eliminating pharmacotherapy right after ending TMS (although the patient was eager to stop her medications now that she was well), and discuss the possibility of retreatment in the event of another episode.

Clinical Vignette

The patient is a 52-year-old man who first received TMS treatment, with a figure-eight coil system, 3 months prior in another state. He reported benefit from TMS, and his records reported a pretreatment PHQ-9 score of 22 and a posttreatment score of 12 (moderate symptoms). He complained that he did not like the length of his previous TMS treatment sessions, which were 50 minutes (he received sequential bilateral treatment), and had concerns about the amount of time he would have to spend away from work. After consultation with his previous TMS physician, he began an on-label course of deep TMS with the H1 coil system; each treatment session was 20 minutes. His pretreatment PHQ-9 score was 18. After he had 20 sessions with a 3-week taper, his posttaper PHQ-9 score was 6.

Clinical Vignette

The patient is a 36-year old woman who was previously treated with TMS at another program after a series of unproductive medication trials. She needed to interrupt that TMS treatment course after only 2 weeks because she went to care for an ill relative who lived in another state. When she returned, she sought treatment with a different TMS system because she had found it difficult to tolerate the earlier treatments ("vibrations with my head inside the machine") and wanted to try a different approach. This time she was treated with a figure-eight ferromagnetic core system and was better able to tolerate the treatments. She had a clinically meaningful improvement in symptoms after 30 treatments at the second facility but fell short of remission. Her health insurer approved additional treatments, requested in an effort to move the patient from response to remission, and she attained remission status after an additional 12 treatments.

Future Directions

Several novel TMS systems are under development and merit some note in this chapter. For the treatment of major depression, two devices under development use low-intensity magnetic fields that do not result in depolarization and action potentials, and another system employs multiple coils with control of the phase relationship between stimulation pulses in the coils. Still other systems are being developed to expand the use of TMS in addition to treatment of depression or to improve its capabilities.

Low-field magnetic stimulation (LFMS; being developed by Tal Medical Inc., Boston, Massachusetts) grew out of the observation that some depressed subjects undergoing magnetic resonance spectroscopy studies reported a mood improvement during the scanning procedure (Rohan et al. 2014). Rather than trains of pulses, the LFMS signal is a trapezoidal magnetic waveform at 500 Hz that generates an electrical field at 1,000 Hz at a low amplitude (<1 V/m) insufficient to cause action potentials. Studies with this system are ongoing.

Synchronized TMS (sTMS) is being developed by NeoSync, Inc. (Newton, Massachusetts). This device generates a low-intensity sinusoidal time-varying magnetic field by rotating sets of neodymium permanent magnets instead of sending an electrical current through a coil. The frequency of the magnetic field is personalized or synchronized to the intrinsic alpha rhythm (on electroencephalogram) of each individual patient (Leuchter et al. 2015). This magnetic field is also below the intensity that will cause action potentials and, as with LFMS, is not targeted at a specific brain region.

Although the five devices with FDA clearance all use a single coil to generate the magnetic field, an alternative approach would be to employ multiple coils that are energized in a phased pattern to direct the magnetic field in ways not attainable with a single, statically positioned coil. The multicoil "steerable" TMS system was initially developed by Cervel Neurotech, Inc. (Redwood City, California), and was acquired in 2015 by Rio Grande Neurosciences, Inc. (Santa Fe, New Mexico). A manuscript describing clinical trial results in major depressive disorder is in submission (L. Carpenter, personal communication, 2016).

Other TMS devices are under development for use outside of the treatment of major depression. Brainsway has reported investigations with deep TMS using a variety of specific coils with different geometries for the treatment of obsessive-compulsive disorder, posttraumatic stress disorder, bipolar depression, and nicotine addiction (Tendler et al. 2016). Neuronix, Ltd. (Yokneam, Israel) is developing a system for use in the treatment of Alzheimer's disease (e.g., Bentwich et al. 2011) in which TMS is combined with cognitive training exercises (ClinicalTrials.gov, NCT01825330). NeuroQore, Inc. (San Francisco, California, and Ottawa, Ontario, Canada) is developing a "monophasic rTMS system," which may have somewhat different physiological effects than those that are generated by the systems with biphasic pulses (NeuroQore Web site, www.neuroqore.com).

Other research efforts span a wide range of refinements that could lead to improved clinical care. One line of work is the development of "patterned TMS," in which pulses are generated in patterns that are more complex, such as theta burst stimulation, than the pulse trains currently employed (Fitzgerald and Daskalakis 2011; Huang et al. 2005). Other developments include the study of potential biomarkers that could predict treatment outcomes of TMS (e.g., Bares et al. 2015; Beuzon et al. 2017; Erguzel et al. 2015); studies of biomarkers could perhaps address important clinical questions, such as who is likely to achieve remission with "conventional" TMS or who would do better with an alternative anatomical target or a different set of stimulation parameters. Still other investigators are exploring the use of neuroimaging data ("neuronavigation") to assist in anatomical targeting (e.g., Beuzon et al. 2017; Rusjan et al. 2010; Schönfeldt-Lecuona et al. 2010; Trojak et al. 2011). Additional scientific research and commercial interest will help to determine which of these additional areas of research may emerge with clinically available and FDA-approved tools.

Conclusion

Neuromodulation techniques represent the "third wave" in psychiatric therapeutics, following the psychotherapies and pharmacotherapies that have dominated mental health care for over a century. TMS stands as a well-tolerated, noninvasive approach to neuromodulation, with strong level 1 evidence to support its clinical efficacy and safety profile. The current set of systems have placed a valuable therapeutic tool in the hands of hundreds of psychiatrists in the United States, who now offer TMS treatment to patients who have struggled with unremitting symptoms and disability for many months if not years.

Many questions remain for which data are lacking. At present, our treatment strategies with TMS are similar to those with medications, in that we start with a set of stimulation parameters and monitor for symptomatic improvement, without a way to match patient to treatment except by empirical trial and error. For example, we will not know how the five FDA-cleared systems compare with each other without comparative effectiveness research trials (Cook et al. 2014), so we do not know if there are some patients who would experience better outcomes with one system or another. Are there some patients who would do best with current on-label treatment parameters (i.e., fast TMS targeted at the left DLPFC) and others who might benefit more from treatment with something that is currently off-label, such as slow, 1-Hz TMS targeted over the right DLPFC? How best might the disabling depressive episodes of bipolar disorder be treated with TMS (see Chapter 8, "Transcranial Magnetic Stimulation for the Treatment of Other Mood Disorders")? What other psychiatric or neurological conditions might benefit from TMS? Our present evidence base, as large as it may be, still leaves many questions unanswered.

As clinical and translational research expands what is known about how magnetic fields modulate the many circuits and systems of the brain, new therapeutic indications and new approaches to stimulation surely will emerge and gain traction. At present, though, the currently cleared devices allow us to successfully treat patients with medication-resistant depression who have not benefited from standard therapeutic options and thereby to restore wellness in many.

KEY CLINICAL POINTS

- Five TMS systems have an FDA clearance (as of February 2017) for use in patients with major depressive disorder who have not responded to one or more antidepressant medications. Four systems employ a figure-eight coil; one system employs an H coil.

- To date there are no head-to-head trials comparing efficacy and safety among these systems. Therefore, TMS referral decisions should consider factors such as quality of care, patient access, and insurance coverage.

- When patients with major depressive disorder are referred for TMS therapy, it is important that the TMS center use an FDA-cleared system that has been approved for use in patients with this disorder.

- New systems are likely to become available in the near future and may offer useful alternatives for delivering care.

References

Advanced Mental Health Care: H-coil types and functionalities. 2012. Available at: AdvancedMentalHealth.com/h-coil-types-and-functionalities. Accessed April 9, 2017.

Avery DH, Isenberg KE, Sampson SM, et al: Transcranial magnetic stimulation in the acute treatment of major depressive disorder: clinical response in an open-label extension trial. J Clin Psychiatry 69(3):441–451, 2008 18294022

Bares M, Brunovsky M, Novak T, et al: QEEG theta cordance in the prediction of treatment outcome to prefrontal repetitive transcranial magnetic stimulation or venlafaxine ER in patients with major depressive disorder. Clin EEG Neurosci 46(2):73–80, 2015 24711613

Barker AT, Jalinous R, Freeston IL: Non-invasive magnetic stimulation of human motor cortex. Lancet 1(8437):1106–1107, 1985 2860322

Bentwich J, Dobronevsky E, Aichenbaum S, et al: Beneficial effect of repetitive transcranial magnetic stimulation combined with cognitive training for the treatment of Alzheimer's disease: a proof of concept study. J Neural Transm (Vienna) 118(3):463–471, 2011 21246222

Beuzon G, Timour Q, Saoud M: Predictors of response to repetitive transcranial magnetic stimulation (rTMS) in the treatment of major depressive disorder. Encephale 43(1):3–9, 2017 28034451

Carpenter LL, Janicak PG, Aaronson ST, et al: Transcranial magnetic stimulation (TMS) for major depression: a multisite, naturalistic, observational study of acute treatment outcomes in clinical practice. Depress Anxiety 29(7):587–596, 2012 22689344

Cohen LG, Roth BJ, Nilsson J, et al: Effects of coil design on delivery of focal magnetic stimulation: technical considerations. Electroencephalogr Clin Neurophysiol 75(4):350–357, 1990 1691084

Cook IA, Espinoza R, Leuchter AF: Neuromodulation for depression: invasive and noninvasive (deep brain stimulation, transcranial magnetic stimulation, trigeminal nerve stimulation). Neurosurg Clin N Am 25(1):103–116, 2014 24262903

Cowey A: The Ferrier Lecture 2004: What can transcranial magnetic stimulation tell us about how the brain works? Philos Trans R Soc Lond B Biol Sci 360(1458):1185–1205, 2005 16147516

Deng ZD, Lisanby SH, Peterchev AV: Electric field depth-focality tradeoff in transcranial magnetic stimulation: simulation comparison of 50 coil designs. Brain Stimulat 6(1):1–13, 2013 22483681

Erguzel TT, Ozekes S, Gultekin S, et al: Neural network based response prediction of rTMS in major depressive disorder using QEEG cordance. Psychiatry Investig 12(1):61–65, 2015 25670947

Fitzgerald PB, Daskalakis ZJ: The effects of repetitive transcranial magnetic stimulation in the treatment of depression. Expert Rev Med Devices 8(1):85–95, 2011 21158543

George MS, Wassermann EM, Williams WA, et al: Daily repetitive transcranial magnetic stimulation (rTMS) improves mood in depression. Neuroreport 6(14):1853–1856, 1995 8547583

Huang YZ, Edwards MJ, Rounis E, et al: Theta burst stimulation of the human motor cortex. Neuron 45(2):201–206, 2005 15664172

Janicak PG, O'Reardon JP, Sampson SM, et al: Transcranial magnetic stimulation in the treatment of major depressive disorder: a comprehensive summary of safety experience from acute exposure, extended exposure, and during reintroduction treatment. J Clin Psychiatry 69(2):222–232, 2008 18232722

Leuchter AF, Cook IA, Feifel D, et al: Efficacy and safety of low-field synchronized transcranial magnetic stimulation (sTMS) for treatment of major depression. Brain Stimulat 8(4):787–794, 2015 26143022

Levkovitz Y, Isserles M, Padberg F, et al: Efficacy and safety of deep transcranial magnetic stimulation for major depression: a prospective multicenter randomized controlled trial. World Psychiatry 14(1):64–73, 2015 25655160

O'Reardon JP, Solvason HB, Janicak PG, et al: Efficacy and safety of transcranial magnetic stimulation in the acute treatment of major depression: a multisite randomized controlled trial. Biol Psychiatry 62(11):1208–1216, 2007 17573044

Pascual-Leone A, Walsh V, Rothwell J: Transcranial magnetic stimulation in cognitive neuroscience—virtual lesion, chronometry, and functional connectivity. Curr Opin Neurobiol 10(2):232–237, 2000 10753803

Rohan ML, Yamamoto RT, Ravichandran CT, et al: Rapid mood-elevating effects of low field magnetic stimulation in depression. Biol Psychiatry 76(3):186–193, 2014 24331545

Roth Y, Zangen A, Hallett M: A coil design for transcranial magnetic stimulation of deep brain regions. J Clin Neurophysiol 19(4):361–370 2002 12436090

Rusjan PM, Barr MS, Farzan F, et al: Optimal transcranial magnetic stimulation coil placement for targeting the dorsolateral prefrontal cortex using novel magnetic resonance image-guided neuronavigation. Hum Brain Mapp 31(11):1643–1652, 2010 20162598

Schönfeldt-Lecuona C, Lefaucheur JP, Cardenas-Morales L, et al: The value of neuronavigated rTMS for the treatment of depression. Neurophysiol Clin 40(1):37–43, 2010 20230934

Tendler A, Barnea Ygael N, Roth Y, et al: Deep transcranial magnetic stimulation (dTMS)—beyond depression. Expert Rev Med Devices 13(10):987–1000, 2016 27601183

Thielscher A, Kammer T: Linking physics with physiology in TMS: a sphere field model to determine the cortical stimulation site in TMS. Neuroimage 17(3):1117–1130, 2002 12414254

Trojak B, Meille V, Chauvet-Gelinier JC, Bonin B: Further evidence of the usefulness of MRI-based neuronavigation for the treatment of depression by rTMS. J Neuropsychiatry Clin Neurosci 23(2):E30–E31, 2011 21677218

Wittich CM, Burkle CM, Lanier WL: Ten common questions (and their answers) about off-label drug use. Mayo Clin Proc 87(10):982–990, 2012 22877654

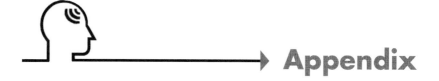

Appendix

Transcranial Magnetic Stimulation Training Courses

All transcranial magnetic stimulation (TMS) device manufacturers provide some degree of on-site introductory training and varying degrees of ongoing support. There are also a growing number of opportunities for advanced training in the form of industry- and nonindustry-sponsored symposia, specialty society courses, and academic medical center courses and fellowships. In addition to providing didactic instruction, some places offer practical hands-on training. Several advanced learning opportunities are listed below.

American Psychiatric Association Annual Meeting (location varies)
Workshops, panel discussions, research presentations
www.psychiatry.org

Berenson-Allen Center for Noninvasive Brain Stimulation
Beth Israel Deaconess Medical Center, Boston, MA
5-day intensive course including hands-on training
http://tmslab.org/education-intensive.php

Clinical TMS Society Annual Meeting (location varies)
Workshops, panel discussions, research presentations
https://clinicaltmssociety.org

Columbia University College of Physicians and Surgeons
Division of Brain Stimulation and Therapeutic Modulation, New
York, NY
5-day intensive course including hands-on training
www.brainstimulation.columbia.edu/education/

Duke University School of Medicine
Department of Psychiatry and Behavioral Sciences, Durham, NC
3-day intensive course including hands-on training
https://psychiatry.duke.edu/course-transcranial-magnetic-stimulation

International Brain Stimulation Conference (location varies)
Symposia, workshops, panel discussions, research presentations,
   hands-on training
www.elsevier.com/events/conferences

International Society for ECT and Neurostimulation Annual Meeting (location varies)
Workshops, panel discussions, research presentations, hands-on
   training
www.isen-ect.org

Medical University of South Carolina
Department of Psychiatry and Behavioral Sciences, Charleston, SC
5-day intensive course including hands-on training
http://academicdepartments.musc.edu/psychiatry/research/bsl/
   Course/

TMS Health Education Advanced Hands-On TMS Symposium
San Francisco, CA
3- or 4-day intensive course with hands-on training
Faculty from various organizations and academic medical centers
http://tmshealtheducation.com

Index

Page numbers printed in **boldface** type refer to tables or figures.